T0292599

A History of Radionuclide Studies in the UK

Ralph McCready • Gopinath Gnanasegaran
Jamshed B. Bomanji
Editors

A History of Radionuclide Studies in the UK

50th Anniversary of the British Nuclear Medicine Society

SIEMENS

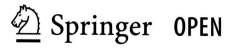 Springer OPEN

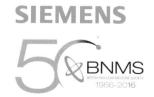

Editors
Ralph McCready
Department of Nuclear Medicine
Royal Sussex County Hospital
Brighton
UK

Jamshed B. Bomanji
Institute of Nuclear Medicine
University College Hospital
London
UK

Gopinath Gnanasegaran
Department of Nuclear Medicine
Guy's and St Thomas' Hospital
London
UK

ISBN 978-3-319-28623-5   ISBN 978-3-319-28624-2   (eBook)
DOI 10.1007/978-3-319-28624-2

Library of Congress Control Number: 2016932527

Printed on acid-free paper

Springer International Publishing AG Switzerland is part of Springer Science+Business Media
(www.springer.com)

Foreword

It is 50 years since a group of pioneering nuclear medicine physicians came together in a Pub in London to discuss how to take nuclear medicine forward in the UK – and the British Nuclear Medicine Society (BNMS) was born. Since the first use of radionuclides for patient treatment in 1948 (using P-32 to treat polycythaemia) and then imaging 1948 (hand-traced maps of thyroid gland), nuclear medicine showed a great potential to unravel the physiological processes in health and disease. During the relatively short 50-year period since the BNMS was founded, there has been immense changes and advances in the speciality: from a scientific curiosity to becoming an indispensable diagnostic and therapeutic tool. The BNMS has been the hub for this highly motivated multidisciplinary group of people which from the start included physicians, scientists, physicists, radio pharmacists, practitioners and nurses. This book is a timely collection of articles outlining the scientific advances in nuclear medicine recorded by the pioneers themselves. This book is a journey through these exciting times, and it is also a collection of personal narratives, telling us the story of these exciting years by those who have themselves been instrumental in advancing and shaping nuclear medicine. I have great pleasure and honour in presenting this book, an informative and an enjoyable read of this journey through five decades of nuclear medicine in the UK, to mark the 50th anniversary of the BNMS.

Nottingham, UK

Alp Notghi

Introduction

The British Nuclear Medicine Society (BNMS) is a registered charity that was originally established in 1966 as the Nuclear Medicine Society. It is the only independent forum devoted to all aspects of nuclear medicine, clinical practice, education, research and development of nuclear medicine within the UK. Nuclear medicine covers the whole spectrum of medical diagnostic, investigational and investigational use of 'unsealed' radionuclides.

The Society is committed to safe practice and high quality standards throughout the UK. As well as co-operating with other professional societies and interested bodies, the BNMS holds two scientific and educational meetings each year around the UK and through its committees, promotes education, good practice, organisational audit and quality assurance activities. The Society provides advice for purchasers on clinical and technical requirements and standards for nuclear medicine as well as responding to NICE when appropriate.

The BNMS also promotes the countrywide audit and quality assurance activities.

Celebrating the 50th Anniversary of the foundation of the BNMS, this booklet brings together the history and scientific achievements in the UK over the past 50 years and more.

Ralph McCready DSc FRCR FRCP Hon FFR RSCI
Jamshed Bomanji MBBS, PhD, FRCR, FRCP
Gopinath Gnanasegaran MD FRCP

Past Presidents of the BNMS

1968/1969	Dr C J Hayter (Leeds)
1969/1970	Prof E M McGirr (Glasgow)
1970/1971	Dr T M D Gimlette (Liverpool)
1971/1972	Prof E S Williams† (London)
1972/1974	Prof R McCready (Sutton)
1974/1976	Prof E Rhys Davies (Bristol)
1976/1978	Dr D Croft (London)
1978/1980	Prof M M Maisey (London)
1980/1982	Dr R F Jewkes (London)
1982/1984	Prof K E Britton (London)
1984/1986	Dr L K Harding (Birmingham)
1986/1988	Prof P S Robinson (Surrey)
1988/1990	Dr A J Coakley (Canterbury)
1990/1992	Prof J H McKillop (Glasgow)
1992/1994	Dr Susan E M Clarke (London)
1994/1996	Dr D H Keeling (Plymouth)
1996/1998	Dr H W Gray (Glasgow)
1998/2000	Dr T O Nunan (London)
2000/2002	Prof P J Robinson (Leeds)
2002/2004	Dr MC Prescott (Manchester)
2004/2006	Dr AJ Hilson (London)
2006/2008	Dr JW Frank (London)
2008/2010	Dr G Vivian (Cornwall)
2010/2012	Prof A C Perkins (Nottingham)
2012/2014	Dr B J Neilly (Glasgow)
2014/2016	Dr Alp Notghi (Birmingham)

Preface

The European Association of Nuclear Medicine (EANM) welcomed in 2015 its 40th National Society and I was very proud, as an EANM member and President, to be present at this symbolic event.

The EANM is based on a broad representation from national societies and more than 3000 individual members, and this mix gives us a particular strength and representation, which is one of the reasons for the success of the EANM. I clearly have in mind the contract that gave birth to the EANM, where two signatures of colleagues from the UK appear. This image well represents the primary role of the British Nuclear Medicine Community in the development of the EANM.

Our European Association turned 25 years old in 2012, quite young when compared to the BNMS, which is celebrating its 50th anniversary!

Both the BNMS and the EANM are lively and well fitted to face the challenges of the modern medical world. Our discipline has unique characteristics and has all the potential to stay as a major player in the clinical and scientific arena.

Many developments have occurred during the life of EANM since its foundation and the British Nuclear Medicine Community has always been active in driving these developments in the best way possible. The British Nuclear Medicine Community has had the privilege to have some of the pioneers of our discipline amongst its members. These scientists contributed to the basis of our discipline in the "old" continent and gave to the European Nuclear Medicine Community the strength that continues to the present day.

Vienna, Austria   Arturo Chiti

Preface

We would like to use this opportunity to congratulate you all on the 50th anniversary of the British Nuclear Medicine Society.

Enhancing the capacity of Member States in the field of nuclear medicine and diagnostic imaging forms an integral part of the International Atomic Energy Agency's objective to accelerate and enlarge the contribution of atomic energy to peace, health and prosperity throughout the world. The unconditional support of British professionals and institutions throughout these 50 years has made a significant contribution to achieving this goal. Provision of training for all disciplines involved in the field and the expertise provided to Member States by British experts has been pivotal in advancing the practice of nuclear medicine and diagnostic imaging worldwide.

Through the generous support of our British colleagues, a total of over 800 trainees have been hosted and over 150 experts have provided their support to countless IAEA Member States. The knowledge and experience shared have enabled professionals to bring nuclear medicine and diagnostic imaging to the forefront on global scale in tackling a variety of diseases, with special emphasis on cardiovascular and cancer diseases. Through our mutual collaboration, we have helped many countries throughout the world to improve the delivery of high-quality practice in a sustainable manner.

We would like to use this opportunity to express our gratitude to the British Nuclear Medicine Society for your support and look forward to future collaboration. We invite you all in your professional or institutional capacities to continue providing support for strengthening the nuclear medicine and diagnostic imaging practice worldwide.

Vienna, Austria

Diana Paez

Contents

Contributors

James R. Ballinger Imaging Sciences, King's College London, London, UK

Lorenzo Biassoni Department of Radiology, Great Ormond Street Hospital for Children NHS Foundation Trust, London, UK

Glen M. Blake Department of Nuclear Medicine, Guy's Campus, King's College London, London, UK

Philip J. Blower Division of Imaging Sciences and Biomedical Engineering, King's College London, St Thomas' Hospital, London, UK

Jamshed Bomanji Clinical Department, Institute of Nuclear Medicine, UCLH NHS Foundation Trust, London, UK

Keith Britton Departments of Radiology and Nuclear Medicine, The London Clinic, London, UK

John Buscombe Department of Nuclear Medicine, Cambridge University Hospitals, Cambridge, UK

Arturo Chiti Humanitas University, Milan, Italy

Humanitas Research Hospital, Milan, Italy

European Association of Nuclear Medicine, Vienna, Austria

Liz Clarke European Applications, GE Healthcare Ltd, The Grove Centre, Amersham, UK

Peter J. Ell Department of Nuclear Medicine, Institute of Nuclear Medicine, UCLH NHS Foundation Trust, London, UK

Ignac Fogelman Department of Nuclear Medicine, Guy's Campus, King's College London, London, UK

Gopinath Gnanasegaran Department Nuclear Medicine, Guy's & St Thomas' NHS Foundation Trust, London, UK

Isky Gordon Great Ormond Street Hospital for Children NHS Foundation Trust, London, UK

Andrew Hilson Department of Nuclear Medicine, Royal Free Hospital, London, UK

Richard S. Lawson Department of Nuclear Medicine, Central Manchester Nuclear Medicine Centre, Salford, UK

University of Salford, Salford, UK

University of Manchester, Manchester, UK

Michael Maisey Kings College, London, UK

Ralph McCready Nuclear Medicine Department, Royal Sussex County Hospital, Brighton, UK

Brian Neilly Department of Nuclear Medicine, Glasgow Royal Infirmary, Glasgow, UK

Alp Notghi Department of Physics and Nuclear Medicine, Sandwell & West Birmingham Hospitals NHS Trust, City Hospital, Birmingham, UK

Tom Nunan Nuclear medicine, St Thomas' Hospital, London, UK

Diana Paez Nuclear Medicine and Diagnostic Imaging Section Division of Human Health Department of Nuclear Sciences and Applications, International Atomic Energy Agency Vienna International Centre, Vienna, Austria

Alan C. Perkins Department of Radiological Sciences, University of Nottingham and Honorary, Nottingham, UK

Nottingham University Hospitals NHS Trust, Nottingham, UK

Michael Peters Department of Nuclear Medicine, Clinical and Laboratory Investigation, Brighton and Sussex Medical School, Brighton, UK

S. Richard Underwood Department Nuclear Medicine, Imperial College London, Royal Brompton Hospital, London, UK

E. David Williams Sunderland, UK

History of the BNMS 1966–2016

Brian Neilly

1.1 Background

The post-war period of the late 1940s and the 1950s was a productive time for developments in the use of radionuclides to diagnose and treat human disease. The pioneers of these developments in the UK were eminent scientists such as Norman Veall, Russell Herbert, WV Mayneord, and John Mallard who carried out research using radiopharmaceuticals and designed and built simple homemade detection systems [1, 2]. The field developed rapidly but failed initially to capture the imagination of clinicians other than endocrinologists such as Edward McGirr (second President of the BNMS) who used 131I to study and treat thyroid disorders. Influenced by progress reported at international meetings, the availability of commercially built scanners and the increasing access to radioisotopes other than I-131, things were changing in the UK and elsewhere. Progress with radioisotopes had largely been the preserve of Medical Physics Departments but by 1960 it was recognised that the move of radioisotopes from bench to bedside necessitated medical leadership of the new discipline of 'Nuclear Medicine', a descriptor imported from North America. The 1960s saw the appointment of the first consultant physicians in Nuclear Medicine in the UK.

1.2 The Original Four

Against this changing landscape, four clinicians with an interest in Nuclear Medicine, Steve Garnett, David Keeling, Ralph McCready and Edward Williams met at the Prince Alfred pub in Queensway, London (Fig. 1.1) on Tuesday 19th July 1966 to

B. Neilly
Department of Nuclear Medicine, Glasgow Royal Infirmary,
Glasgow G31 2ER, UK

© The Author(s) 2016
R. McCready et al. (eds.), *A History of Radionuclide Studies in the UK:
50th Anniversary of the British Nuclear Medicine Society*,
DOI 10.1007/978-3-319-28624-2_1

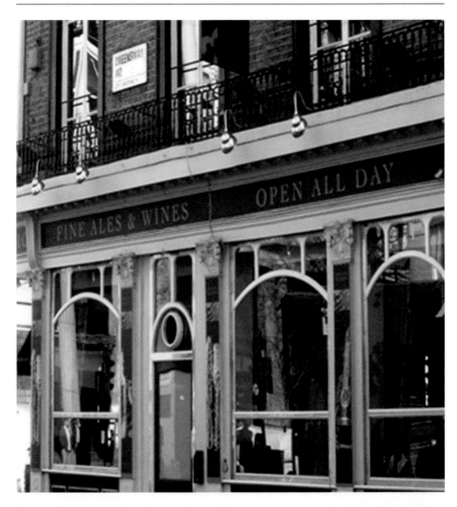

Fig. 1.1 The Prince Alfred, Queensway, London

discuss the future professional situation of physicians working in Nuclear Medicine [2]. The group formed the Nuclear Medicine Society (NMS) and resolved to hold 4 meetings a year. This was a courageous move leaving behind, as they did, the protective environment of more established medical associations. The NMS meetings were held initially at the Middlesex Hospital, London and took the form of evening meetings followed by a buffet supper. Initially there were no officers but Ralph McCready took on the role as Secretary and David Keeling produced a short newsletter. The first AGM was held in December 1966 and the rules and byelaws were agreed and approved at a meeting of the NMS at the Middlesex Hospital on 6th October 1967. The first formal election of NMS officers took place in December 1967. Clive Hayter (Leeds) was elected as first President, Ralph McCready was confirmed as the Honorary Secretary and Steve Garnett (Southampton) as Treasurer. At this time the fledgling society numbered 25 members and in January 1968 subscriptions were levied at £1 increasing to £2 by October of that year. In recognition of the many national Nuclear Medicine specialist groups that had formed globally, an EGM was convened on 19 November 1969, and the meeting voted to change its name from the 'Nuclear Medicine Society' to the 'British Nuclear Medicine Society' (BNMS) [3].

1.3   First Steps

By the late 1960s interest in Nuclear Medicine in the UK was growing fast and in June 1969 the Royal College of Physicians held a meeting entitled 'Advances in the Application of Physics in Medicine' incorporating advances in Nuclear Medicine. The May 1970 BNMS Newsletter gave details of the London University Nuclear Medicine MSc course that commenced later that year. In 1971, Edward Williams, then head of the Institute of Nuclear Medicine at the Middlesex Hospital, was elected BNMS President and the same year became the first UK Professor of Nuclear Medicine. A paper given by Edward Williams at the 'Whither Nuclear Medicine' meeting at the Royal College of Surgeons in Lincoln's Field in May 1971 helped foster the association with internal medicine. By 1972 there were 140 rectilinear scanners in the UK and 30 gamma cameras, a remarkable advance given that the first UK commercial scanner had been installed in 1958 at the Royal Marsden [3] The success of clinical Nuclear Medicine highlighted tensions between the various professional bodies involved in Nuclear Medicine in the UK particularly over the matter of the HPA document 'Organisation of Hospital Radioisotope Services (Nuclear Medicine) in the UK' [3]. These difficulties were resolved by discussion and the groups have continued to work collaboratively over the years. Important associations were formed early on between the BNMS and international organisations such as the World Federation of Nuclear Medicine and Biology (WFNMB). In 1971 the BNMS was invited to sign as the UK representative to the WFNMB. In June 1974, Desmond Croft attended the ENMS meeting at Clermont-Ferrand and signed up the BNMS as the specialist NM society representing the UK [3]. Such developments helped strengthen and establish the BNMS as the recognised professional organisation devoted to Nuclear Medicine in the UK.

1.4   Annual Meetings

By the early 1970s efforts were concentrated on the creation of an annual meeting and AGM. The first annual meeting of the BNMS took place in 1973 in the Windeyer Building at the Middlesex Hospital and included a small commercial exhibition [4]. By 1975, and for economic reasons, the annual meeting [3] was held at the University of London Student's union in Malet Street where the registration fee was £1 (£2 for non-members). The 1976 annual meeting was a 2-day conference held in association with the HPA where 24 proffered papers were presented [5]. The 1978 BNMS annual meeting was held jointly with the ENMS and SNME (the forerunner organisations of the EANM) prompting a move to Imperial College where the venue remained until 1995. The single exception to this was 1985 (the year of the joint ENMS/SNME/BNMS meeting at the Barbican) when a 1-day BNMS meeting was held at the University of Manchester Institute of Science and Technology during April. The 1980 annual meeting was the first UK meeting to be held over 3 days. The newsletter commented that one of the strengths of the meeting was 'the enthusiasm of the commercial exhibitors to display and discuss their wares' [6]. By 1986 at the 14th annual meeting, there were 162 proffered papers of which 119 were accepted and it was generally agreed that the standard of the scientific papers was high [5]. A central feature of the annual meeting is the guest lecture. Of the many distinguished lectures over the years, the BNMS were honoured to have Professor Henry Wagner deliver the 1987 guest lecture entitled 'Imaging the Chemistry of Mental Illness.'

The need for space to accommodate the commercial exhibition necessitated a move away from Imperial College to more suitable venues. In 1996 the annual meeting was held in Brighton and thereafter at various venues including Brighton, Manchester and Edinburgh until 2009. The delegate numbers peaked at 768 at Brighton in 2000. However, the spiralling costs of the larger centres meant that it was no longer financially viable to continue at large city venues and a decision was taken to alternate between Harrogate and Brighton where the venue hire was more affordable during the period 2009–2015. The 2016 Annual Meeting will be held in Birmingham where fittingly the President is Dr Alp Notghi.

1.5   Joint Meetings with EANM

Since its formation, the BNMS has held four joint meetings with the EANM in the UK. These were in 1978 at Imperial College, 1985 at the Barbican Centre, 1997 at the SECC Glasgow and 2011 at the ICC Birmingham. Over 3,000 delegates attended the Barbican Centre in 1985 where the Congress President was Keith Britton and the BNMS President was Keith Harding. The Congress President at the Glasgow Meeting in 1997 was Jim McKillop and the BNMS President was Harry Gray. Over 5,400 participants attended the 2011 Birmingham meeting where the local organiser was Alan Perkins, the first non-medical President of the BNMS.

1.6   Membership

As a registered charity the BNMS is the only independent multi-disciplinary professional forum in the UK devoted to all aspects of Nuclear Medicine. The Board of Trustees of the BNMS (known as the Council) is responsible for the charity. Its members include clinical scientists, nuclear medicine physicians, nurses, radiologists, radiopharmacists and technologists. Initially, full membership of the BNMS was open only to medically qualified persons although Council had the right to admit to membership individuals thought to have a valid claim. At the AGM in 1972 the rules and byelaws were changed to allow non-medical colleagues to become full members of the BNMS [3]. As an means of widening membership further, the Charities Commission was approached and gave permission in 1980 to establish a new category entitled 'associate membership' open to all scientists, pharmacists, technicians and medical staff not eligible for full membership. The initial associate membership fee was set at £8 allowing access to the newsletter section of the journal and reduced fees at BNMS meetings [3]. As a result of this and reflecting the growing interest in Nuclear Medicine, BNMS membership increased from 220 in 1982 to 752 (including 195 associate members) in the year 2000. The membership numbers have subsequently decreased but fluctuate between 450 and 500 members at present. The growth of the BNMS necessitated a change to the legal status of the organisation and in 2012 following a successful application to Companies House, the BNMS was incorporated under the Companies Act 2006 as a company limited by guarantee.

1.7   Aims and Objectives

While the agenda of early BNMS council meetings was dominated of necessity by the formation of its rules and byelaws and the arrangement of its scientific meetings, the matters discussed by council included issues of national concern such as staff training (technical and medical), advice to government bodies on the registration, authorisation and safe use of radioisotopes in medicine, and collaboration with other professional organisations such as HPA and BIR [3]. The business of these first BNMS Council meetings helped shape the aims and objectives of the Society that were subsequently crystallised and set out in the Articles of Association and now captured in the BNMS strategic plan 2010–2013 [7]. To help Council achieve its objectives, there are a number of Committees or Groups that report to Council. These include Professional Standards, Education, Science, Research & Innovation, Public Relations, Therapy and PET-CT groups. The administrative functions of the BNMS were ably supported by a number of individuals but notably by Sue Hatchard who was administrative secretary between 1986 until 2013. Sue ran the BNMS from the office in Regent House, SE London and on her retiral, the BNMS Offices moved to the Jubilee Campus at Nottingham University where Charlotte Weston is the Chief Executive Officer.

1.8   The Journal

A significant development for Nuclear Medicine in general and the BNMS in particular was the creation of Nuclear Medicine Communications. The journal was formed to facilitate rapid communication of information within the international community. The first issue of Nuclear Medicine Communications was published in 1980 in association with the BNMS [8]. The success story that is Nuclear Medicine and the part played by the BNMS in its remarkable progress in the UK can be seen in the pages of NMC, as well as at scientific meetings of the BNMS and on its webpages.

References

1. Schicha H, Bergdolt K, Ell PJ, editors. History of Nuclear Medicine in Europe. Stuttgart/New York: Schatthauer; 2003. p. 75–9.
2. McCready RV. History of the British Nuclear Medicine Society. http://www.bnms.org.uk/images/stories/History/EANM_25_Anniversary_UK.pdf.
3. Keeling D. Historical notes on the first 10 years (unpublished observations).
4. McCready RV. 40th anniversary BNMS annual meeting. http://www.bnms.org.uk/images/stories/History/history_poster.pdf.
5. Harding LK. British Nuclear Medicine Society 14th annual meeting. Nucl Med Commun. 1986;7:209–10.
6. Editorial. BNMS Newsletter. Nucl Med Commun 1980;1(3):147–52.
7. BNMS strategic plan 2010–2013. http://www.bnms.org.uk/images/stories/Official_Documents/BNMS_Strat_plan_Final_2011.pdf.
8. Britton K. Editorial. Nucl Med Commun 1980;(1):1–2.

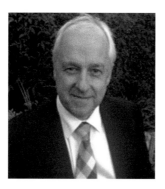

Brian Neilly I graduated MB ChB from the University of Dundee and completed my house jobs with Dr Robert Fife in Medicine and with Professor David Carter in Surgery at Glasgow Royal Infirmary (GRI). I was offered a post in surgery but preferred the physician route and joined the medical SHO rotation at GRI and completed the MRCP examination. A medical registrar post followed during which I completed research for my MD in Cor Pulmonale after which I undertook a research fellowship in sleep medicine at the University of Pennsylvania in Philadelphia. On my return to the UK I was appointed Senior Registrar in Internal Medicine and Nuclear Medicine at GRI where my training was with two former Presidents of the BNMS, Professor Jim McKillop and Dr Harry Gray of the University Medical Unit. I was appointed Consultant Physician with an interest in Nuclear and Respiratory Medicine at Glasgow Royal Infirmary in 1995 and, being a physician at heart, still enjoy the challenge of the acute medical take and continuing care of ward patients. Due to my interest in Nuclear Medicine training I have held posts as Chair of the STC, SAC and ICSCNM and am external examiner to the London Nuclear Medicine MSc. In line with my continued interest in pulmonary embolism, I was a co-author of the EANM Guidelines on VQ SPECT in Pulmonary Embolism 2009. As President of the BNMS from 2012 to 2014 I was lead author of the Medical Radioisotopes Report 2014. As Chair of the ICSCNM I led the successful initiative to apply to the GMC for Curriculum Change in Nuclear Medicine Training in the UK, commenced 2015.

Brian Neilly MB ChB MD FCRP (Glasgow & London) FRCR

My thanks to Ralph McCready, Andrew Hilson, Harry Gray and of course the notes by David Keeling on the first 10 years, for providing detail on the historical background of the BNMS.

A History of Nuclear Medicine in the UK

2

Ralph McCready

The use of radioisotopes in the UK can be traced from the first tracer study carried out by George von Hevesy. Von Hevesy was born in Hungary studied in Germany and came to work with Ernest Rutherford in Manchester in 1911. His task was to separate Radium D from lead. He suspected that his landlady was reusing food left on his dinner plate. He put some ^{212}Pb into the left overs and some days later used a radiation detector to detect it confirming that his landlady was in fact recycling his food (Fig. 2.1).

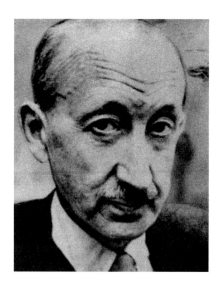

Fig. 2.1 Georges von Hevesy

R. McCready
Nuclear Medicine Department, Royal Sussex County Hospital,
Brighton BN2 5BE, UK

© The Author(s) 2016
R. McCready et al. (eds.), *A History of Radionuclide Studies in the UK:
50th Anniversary of the British Nuclear Medicine Society*,
DOI 10.1007/978-3-319-28624-2_2

The early use of radionuclides in the UK was hindered by the McMahon Act in the US prohibiting the export of radioisotopes made in reactors until 1947. However as one of the peaceful uses of atomic energy UK government money was being poured into the Atomic Energy Research Establishment at Harwell to produce radioisotopes. Already in 1947 J S Mitchell listed most of the radioisotopes that would be used as tracers. The first isotope conference sponsored by Harwell was held in Oxford in 1951 Fig. 2.2 [1]. By 1954 colloidal gold bismuth 206 and phosphorus were being produced for therapy and iodine 131 iron 59 chromium 51 for human diagnostic procedures. With the support of the Medical Research Council medical radioisotope units managed by physicists were being formed. At the Hammersmith Hospital the first therapeutic dose of P-32 was used in November 1947 to treat a young girl with a glioma [1, 2]. By 1954 Professor Sir David Smithers at the Royal Cancer Hospital London listed treatments on 96 patients using ^{32}P, ^{131}I, ^{24}Na, ^{82}Br, and ^{198}Au [3]. The non-therapeutic use of radioisotopes concentrated primarily on human physiology. In 1957 John West studied lung perfusion with oxygen-15 produced by the first recently installed cyclotron at the MRC unit at the Hammersmith Hospital. Other in vitro studies included those on whole body water, blood volume and red cell turnover, calcium metabolism, cardiac and renal function.

The original reference book was that of Veall and Vetter 1958 entitled Radioisotopes in Clinical Research and Diagnosis (later edited by Belcher and Vetter). Counting was done using home-made circuitry with Geiger Counters. Norman Veall devised a circular array of Geiger counters to count urine in a

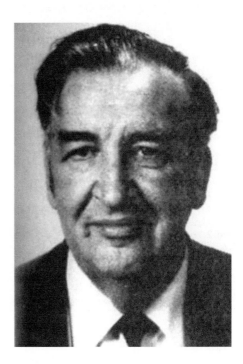

Fig. 2.2 Norman Veall

Winchester bottle. These were eventually replaced by scalers and ratemeters made by E K Cole in Southend and Isotope Developments Ltd Aldermaston which later became part of Nuclear Enterprises Edinburgh. Norman Veall is remembered by the Norman Veall medal presented to a clinical scientist annually at the BNMS.

A key development of in vitro studies in the UK was made by Roger Ekins at the Middlesex Hospital London who in 1960 enabled the quantitative determination of thyroid hormones in blood samples using radioactive isotopes and specific binding proteins [4]. Radioactive B 12 was produced by J M Bradley at the Hammersmith Hospital with high specific activity cobalt-56 with the help of Glaxo. Direct evidence of B 12 absorption in the ileum in 1959 by found by Booth and Mollin who studied the distribution of radioactivity in the intestine after oral administration of radio labelled B 12. using a Geiger counter during a laparotomy [5].

In 1949 Ansell and Rotblat in Liverpool made the first radioisotope image in the UK of a patient with a retrosternal goiter [6]. By 1955 the precursor of imaging used hand held Geiger counters to plot iso-contours of iodine 131 activity in the thyroid gland. Russell Herbert also in Liverpool used a small calcium half inch diameter tungstate crystal on an early photo multiplier tube to improve the sensitivity. Early single and multibore lead collimators improved the resolution.

An early scintillation detector designed for brain studies with Iodine 131 fluorescein was made in March 1951 by Belcher and Evans at the Royal Cancer Hospital (now the Royal Marsden Hospital) in London. The photomultiplier tube had to be cooled by liquid nitrogen to reduce the background noise. To avoid the possibility of frostbite, the patient's skin and the crystal were separated by a long Perspex light guide!

Also in 1951 rectilinear scanning was being developed to make iodine 131 thyroid imaging easier. The first device in the UK was made at the Royal Cancer Hospital London in 1951 to image initially radionuclide sources and then the thyroid gland. The Mayneord scanner displayed images on a Cathode Ray Tube, used Geiger counters, collimator, background subtraction and a clever raster scanning mechanism (Fig. 2.3).

Reprinted from Radioisotope Techniques. Vol. I, Medical and Physiological Applications (Proceedings of the Isotope Techniques Conference, Oxford, July 1951). (Published by H.M. Stationery Office, price £2 10s. 0d. net, by post £2 11s. 0d.)

A method of making visible the distribution of activity in a source of ionizing radiation[1]

by W. V. MAYNEORD, R. C. TURNER, S. P. NEWBERY and H. J. HODT

Physics Department, Royal Cancer Hospital, London, S.W.3

Fig. 2.3 A copy of the paper by Mayneord et al. of the first UK radioisotope scanner presented at the 1st Harwell sponsored Oxford conference in 1951

The scanner was preceded in 1950 by that shown by Ziedes des Plantes at the London International Radiological Congress [7]. Benedict Cassen in the US also published his paper on a thyroid scanner in Nucleonics 1951.

Professor Val Mayneord inventor of the first UK radioisotope scanner and his wife Audrey met with Professor Ian Donald inventor of the ultrasound scanning in the Nuclear Medicine and Ultrasound Department at the Royal Marsden Hospital in Sutton Fig. 2.4.

The first home made whole body scanner with a colour print out was built in 1957 at the Hammersmith Hospital by Mallard and Peachey [8]. Also home-made was the first UK digital whole body SPECT scanner in Aberdeen. The first commercial Tri-D scanner was installed in the Royal Marsden Hospital Sutton in 1963. It lacked adequate collimation and soon after a 3″ Picker rectilinear scanner was purchased. In the days before ultrasound I-131 labeled albumin was used to

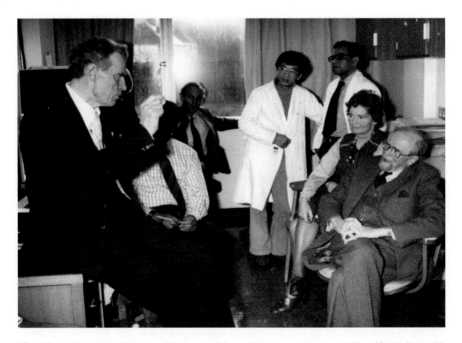

Fig. 2.4 Professor Val Mayneord inventor of the radioisotope scanner and his wife Audrey with Professor Ian Donald inventor of ultrasound scanning. In the background is Professor Kit Hill, Head of the joint department of Medical Physics Institute of Cancer Research and Royal Marsden Hospital Sutton

Fig. 2.5 A photoscan of abdomen showing the placenta taken with a 3″ Picker Magnascanner using I-131 labeled albumin

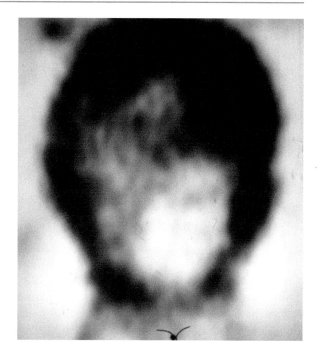

demonstrate the position of the placenta! Fig. 2.5. Those were the days in which anything was possible. The burdensome legislation governing the use of radioactivity was yet to come.

In the mid 1960s Glass and Westerman installed the UK's first Anger Gamma Camera at the Hammersmith.

A local firm Ekco Electronics Ltd in Southend constructed an Anger type gamma camera in 1964 using 9 photomultipler tubes and a 5 in. cryatal. It was not a great commercial success.

In 1977 another local firm J&P constructed the first UK tomoscanner with the assistance of David Keeling and Andrew Todd-Pokropek. It was placed in the Middlesex Hospital London for evaluation. Tl 201 scans using it were published in 1979 from the UK and France.

In the early days of renography Marcus Hall a radiotherapist at Canterbury Hospital developed a technique to eliminate blood background activity [9]. A computerized version of this technique was later developed by Britton and Brown in 1970.

1967 was a good year for innovation. The first paper using F-18 produced by the MRC cyclotron unit for rectilinear scans of bone showed a massive improvement in sensitivity from strontium-89 was published in 1967. With a half life of 109.8 min

Fig. 2.6 Se-75 methionine pancreatic scan imaged on an Intertechnique computer

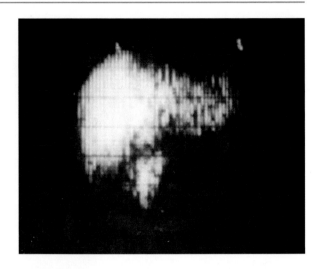

it was fortunate that the traffic flow and the number of traffic lights between Hammermith and Royal Marsden in Sutton was quite low [10]. In the same year Norman Veall published with Steve Garnett the still used technique for the measurement of Glomerular Filtration Rate [11]. Initially devised to improve tumour detection in brain scanning a ratio subtract device was constructed in the physics workshop in the Institute of Cancer Research in Sutton Surrey in 1967 [12]. Later the device was used to eliminate the liver uptake of seleno-methionine in pancreas scanning [13]. The same technique was performed on an early digital computer by Intertechnique Fig. 2.6. It is interesting to reflect on how exciting such awful images were. In fact this was a good example since many pancreas images consisted of about 15 dots.

In 1969 Roy Parker with his colleagues from the Atomic Weapons Research Establishment developed the first semiconductor camera [14]. Using a cooled germanium detector clear images of a rat's tiny thyroid were shown at an IAEA Medical Radioisotope Scintigraphy meeting in Vienna long before the invention of the current solid state cameras. Kromek in the UK is currently advancing CZT technology to provide similar high resolution solid state SPECT camera imaging without the need for cooling.

Fazio and Jones at the Hammersmith reported in 1975 on the use of the generator produced 13 s half life [81m]Kr for gamma camera imaging of regional lung ventilation. The 190 Kev gamma ray emission complimented [99m]Tc 140 Kev emission there by enabling simultaneous ventilation; perfusion imaging. The [81]Rb/[81m]Kr generator was developed by Clark and Watson who responded to the demand for this 4.7 h half-life generator across the UK. As a result at one point [81m]Kr/ [99m]Tc based ventilation: perfusion imaging was the second most frequent imaging procedure in the UK after ^{99m}Tc bone scanning.

As the krypton generator was delivered to the individual hospitals only once or twice per week it was important for patients to have their suspected pulmonary embolus on those days only! 1977 saw the first use of I-123 hippuran for gamma camera renography by O'Reilly and colleagues in Manchester [15].

Following the demonstration of dopamine receptors in the brain by Henry Wagner in 1983 Imaging Dopamine Receptors in the Human Brain by Positron Tomography using 3-N-[^{11}C]methylspiperone. Steve Garnett et al. who had left Guys Hospital for McMaster Canada had imaged F18 fluoro-dopa with their home built brain PET scanner to show the distribution of dopamine in the basal ganglia published in Nature in 1983 and John Crawley in the UK demonstrated dopamine receptors in human brain with 77Br-p-bromospiperone the benefit of Br-77 being its 57 h half life [16]. In 1985 Peter Ell and his colleagues at the Middlesex Hospital published the world first cerebral blood flow image using the Amersham produced Tc99m labeled HM-PAO [17].

In the early 1980s, studies with the UK's first commercial PET scanner at the MRC's Cyclotron Unit at Hammersmith demonstrated the Warburg effect of anaerobic glycolysis of human tumors by showing that gliomas preferred to metabolize glucose (^{18}FDG) to oxygen (^{15}O). It was also reported for the first time by Nolop that lung tumors have a high uptake of ^{18}FDG. This set the scene for the introduction of clinical PET world-wide where ^{18}FDG Lung cancer PET imaging was the first procedure to be reimbursed in the USA. Also the enhanced uptake of ^{18}FDG in breast cancer was reported by Beaney at that time. It should also be noted that the first use of FDG was in the UK by Bessel et al. who explored its use as an anti-cancer agent [18]

The introduction of Sr-89 by Amersham International (Metastron) led to a study of a treatment for painful bone metastases from prostate cancer by the Southampton Group in 1991. A randomized trial of 32 patients showed the benefit of the treatment against stable strontium [19]. In 2002 a grant from the National Institutes of Health enabled the Royal Marsden/Institute of Cancer Research group to test the feasibility and toxicity of high activities of Rhenium-186 hydroxyethylidene diphosphonate, with peripheral blood stem cell rescue in patients with progressive hormone refractory prostate cancer metastatic to bone [20]. It was hoped that the high activities would ablate the metastases as well as relieving bone pain. The long term results of that study are being evaluated.

More recently in 2013 the Royal Marsden published a multicentre Phase 3 study on the use of Re-223 for the palliation of bone pain on the effect on overall survival from metastases from castration resistant prostate cancer. The result showed a significant improvement on overall survival [21].

The first administration of radioiodine for thyroid cancer in the UK was given by Sir Eric Pochin in 1949. While the results from the use of radioiodine thyroid cancer have been excellent as early as 1964 Pochin was already recording untoward side effects from its use. There remains controversy on the balance between giving high activities to ensure total eradication of any residual disease and giving low activities to minimize the risks and shorten isolation in the hospital.

A first UK wide randomised HiLo study compared the effectiveness of 30 and 90 mCi of I-131 for post operative ablation of residual thyroid tissue. In the paper published in the New England Journal of Medicine in 2012 the results of the HiLo study opened the possibility of a complete change in practice reducing the post operative ablative administered activity [22]. Following the success of that trial a new UK nation-wide study comparing the administration of Iodine 131 with none in low risk patients is being carried out.

The UK can be proud of its long record of the development of radionuclide studies. Its input has ranged from the introduction of new radionuclides and techniques, the development of new equipment, and the use of radionuclides in a wide variety of diseases. It is fortunate that the innovation and research continues with the development at Kings of Ga-68 compounds which should widen the use of high resolution PET imaging both in the number of applications and its spread to centres distant from the cyclotrons.

References

1. Mitchell JS. Applications of recent advances in nuclear physics to medicine; with special reference to the pile and the cyclotron as sources of radioactive isotopes. Br J Radiol. 1946;19(228):481–7.
2. Mallard J, Trott NG. Some aspects of the history of nuclear medicine in the United Kingdom. Semin Nucl Med. 1979;9(3):203–17.
3. Smithers DW. Some varied applications of radioactive isotopes to the localization and treatment of tumors. Acta Radiol. 1951;35(1):49–61.
4. Ekins R. Direct determination of free thyroxin in undiluted serum by equilibrium dialysis/radioimmunoassay. Clin Chem. 1989;35(3):510–2.
5. Booth CC, MOLLIN DL. The site of absorption of vitamin B12 in man. Lancet. 1959;1(7062):18–21.
6. Ansell G, Rotblat J. Radioactive iodine as a diagnostic aid for intrathoracic goitre. 1948. Br J Radiol. 1995;68(810):H121–7.
7. B G Ziedses des Plantes. Direct and Indirect autoradiography, Proceedings 6th International Congress of Radiology. London. 1950; p 172.
8. Mallard JR, Peachey CJ. A quantitative automatic body scanner for the localisation of radioisotopes in vivo. Br J Radiol. 1959;32:652–7.
9. Hall FM, Monks GK. The renogram. A method of separating vascular and renal components. Invest Radiol. 1966;1(3):220–4.
10. French RJ, McCready VR. The use of 18-F for bone scanning. Br J Radiol. 1967;40(477):655–61.
11. Garnett ES, Parsons V, Veall N. Measurement of glomerular filtration-rate in man using a 51Cr-edetic-acid complex. Lancet. 1967;1(7494):818–9.
12. Burn GP, Cottrall MF, Field EO. A ratio-subtract device for detecting selective localisation of isotopes in clinical scintiscanning. Br J Radiol. 1967;40(469):62–5.
13. McCready VR, Cottrall MF. Combined pancreas and liver scanning using a double isotope technique. Br J Radiol. 1971;44(527):870–7.

14. McCready VR, Parker RP, Gunnersen EM, Ellis R, Moss E, Gore WG, et al. Clinical tests on a prototype semiconductor gamma-camera. Br J Radiol. 1971;44(517):58–62.
15. O'Reilly PH, Herman KJ, Lawson RS, Shields RA, Testa HJ. 123-Iodine: a new isotope for functional renal scanning. Br J Urol. 1977;49(1):15–21.
16. Crawley JC, Smith T, Veall N, Zanelli GD, Crow TJ, Owen F. Dopamine receptors displayed in living human brain with 77Br-p-bromospiperone. Lancet. 1983;2(8356):975.
17. Ell PJ, Jarritt PH, Cullum I, Hocknell JM, Costa DC, Lui D, et al. Regular cerebral blood flow mapping with 99mTc-labelled compound. Lancet. 1985;2(8445):50–1.
18. Bessell EM, Courtenay VD, Foster AB, Jones M, Westwood JH. Some in vivo and in vitro antitumour effects of the deoxyfluoro-D-glucopyranoses. Eur J Cancer. 1973;9(7):463–70.
19. Lewington VJ, McEwan AJ, Ackery DM, Bayly RJ, Keeling DH, Macleod PM, et al. A prospective, randomised double-blind crossover study to examine the efficacy of strontium-89 in pain palliation in patients with advanced prostate cancer metastatic to bone. Eur J Cancer. 1991;27(8):954–8.
20. O'Sullivan JM, McCready VR, Flux G, Norman AR, Buffa FM, Chittenden S, et al. High activity Rhenium-186 HEDP with autologous peripheral blood stem cell rescue: a phase I study in progressive hormone refractory prostate cancer metastatic to bone. Br J Cancer. 2002;86(11):1715–20.
21. Parker C, Nilsson S, Heinrich D, Helle SI, O'Sullivan JM, Fossa SD, et al. Alpha emitter radium-223 and survival in metastatic prostate cancer. N Engl J Med. 2013;369(3):213–23.
22. Mallick U, Harmer C, Yap B, Wadsley J, Clarke S, Moss L, et al. Ablation with low-dose radioiodine and thyrotropin alfa in thyroid cancer. N Engl J Med. 2012;366(18):1674–85.

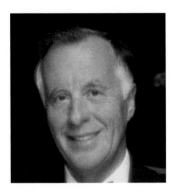

Ralph McCready I graduated from Queens University Belfast with a BSc in Physiology and my medical degree. As a houseman I worked in the Royal Victoria Hospital for Dr Frank Pantridge who invented the defibrillator. I was fascinated by his catheter laboratory and decided to study physiology in radiology. I moved to Guy's Hospital London to study for an MSc in Radiation Physics and Biology together with a Diploma in Medical Radiological Diagnosis (DMRD). My next position was an S.H.O in the Radiology Department of the Hammersmith Hospital where I used to assist Professor Steiner at the beginning of interventional radiology. During a locum in the newly opened Royal Marsden Hospital in Sutton I was offered a research position in the Institute of Cancer Research in the Isotope Unit by Dr E.O. Field. Early publications included mediastinal lymph node scanning in 1967 and F-18 imaging of bone metastases also in 1967.

Eventually I became a Consultant in Nuclear Medicine in charge of the Nuclear Medicine and Ultrasound Department for over 40 years. With Nuclear Medicine and the Medical Physics departments at either end of the same corridor I was fortunate to be able to take part in many projects involving innovations in nuclear medicine, ultrasound equipment magnetic resonance spectroscopy and radiopharmacy. It was privilege to work with Nigel Trott, Bob Ott and Maggie Flower, Martin Leach, Kit Hill and Glenn Flux amongst others. In 1973 I was awarded the Barclay Prize by the British Institute of Radiology for my contributions to the British Journal of Radiology. I was awarded a DSc in the Faculty of Science of Queens University in 1987. In 1974 I was elected to a Fellowship of the Royal College of Physicians London and in 1975 was conferred a Fellow of the Royal College of Radiologists London. I was conferred an Honorary Fellowship of the Faculty of Radiologists, Royal College of Surgeons, Ireland in 1992 and in 2004 was made an Honorary Member of the Japanese Radiological Society. In 1978 I was a vice president of the European Nuclear Medicine Society the chairman of the task group on Education and Training of the EANM 1988–1991 which preceded the European School of Nuclear Medicine.

Now retired I still enjoy publishing and presenting at National and International meetings. I am a Professor Emeritus at the Institute of Cancer Research London and an Honorary Consultant at the Royal Sussex County Hospital in Brighton, U.K.

The Evolution of Training in Nuclear Medicine in the UK

3

Andrew Hilson

Training in Nuclear Medicine in the UK has evolved over the years. This memoire is a personal view, based on a (fallible) memory and documents kept over the years.

It was in the late 1960s that physicians became involved in the developing speciality, which had been predominantly a development of the strong Medical Physics community. A key driver was the creation of the Institute of Nuclear Medicine at the Middlesex Hospital. A particular leader was Professor Edward Williams.

There was much discussion before the MSc was set up as an Intercollegiate Exam of London University. Several Nuclear Medicine physicians felt that the a degree was too rigid, and that there should be a diploma of the Royal College of Physicians (RCP) Other specialties had Diplomas – there was the DObs in Obstetrics, the DA in anaesthetics, the DMRD in radiology, and the DTMH in tropical medicine amongst many. However the Colleges were trying to get rid of Diplomas, so the MSc it was.

In 1971, there was a joint meeting of the British Institute of Radiology, the British Nuclear Medicine Society, the Faculty of Radiologists, the Hospital Physicists' Association and the Section of Radiology of The Royal Society of Medicine, held at The Royal College of Surgeons, Lincoln's Inn Fields, on Friday, May 21,1971 [1]. The Chairman was Dr. James Bull (Senior Radiologist at the National Hospital for Nervous Diseases). The title was "Whither Nuclear Medicine ?" This looked at the provision of Nuclear Medicine services in the light of the Windeyer Report (Report of the Working Party on the Organization of Radioisotope Services, 1970) set up in 1966. Edward Williams gave a paper on "The training programme of future medical Consultants and staff of nuclear medicine departments" in which he proposed that the UK should follow Australia and consider Nuclear Medicine as a specialty which belonged in internal medicine, rather than radiology.

A. Hilson
Department of Nuclear Medicine, Royal Free Hospital, London NW3 2QG, UK

© The Author(s) 2016
R. McCready et al. (eds.), *A History of Radionuclide Studies in the UK:*
50th Anniversary of the British Nuclear Medicine Society,
DOI 10.1007/978-3-319-28624-2_3

Desmond Croft from St Thomas's Hospital was the RCP representative on the UEMS, and thanks to him Nuclear Medicine was recognised as a separate specialty.

When I started on the MSc in 1974, the course was a 2-year course if taken part-time (which is what UK trainees did), or 1 year for overseas students – the majority. The clinical part of the course was taught via the Institute of Nuclear Medicine, and the science via the department of Medical Physics at the Royal Free Hospital School of Medicine, which had smart new teaching facilities in the new hospital in Hampstead (the RFHSM was the only London medical school which accepted candidates without A-level physics, who then had to take a 1st MB course). The resources included a neutron source – one of the practicals I remember involved producing a short-lived isotope by neutron activation then calculating its half-life.

There were lectures on PET – I remember thinking that this would never take off.

Nuclear Medicine in those days included much more in-vitro work, and I remember seeing with relief that one of the questions in the written paper involved giving a full account of an in-vitro assay. That was simple for me – I had set up and ran an assay for Human Placental Lactogen (HPL) – a hormone found in the blood during pregnancy, whose level fell about 2 weeks before birth (this was before obstetric ultrasound).

The dissertation had to be typed – I still have my copy with the text getting fainter as the ribbon wore out.

In 1993 I became an Examiner for the London University Intercollegiate Course for the M.Sc. in Nuclear Medicine, and in 1994 Chairman of the Board of Examiners.

In 1999 Manchester was approved as a teaching centre – prior to that, students had to be attached to a London centre.

In the same year the MSc underwent a major change. London University decided that it didn't want to organise and validate intercollegiate courses, such as the MSc in Nuclear Medicine. There was again discussion about a possible College diploma, but this was even less popular. The Institute of Nuclear Medicine was unable to take over the whole course, so in 2000 the MSc moved to King's College London School of Medicine (KCL). This involved a massive amount of paperwork as the course was remodelled to comply with their regulations. This was mainly undertaken by Drs Sue Clarke and Muriel Buxton-Thomas.

I continued as Chairman of the Board of Examiners, but at short notice KCL said that the post had to be occupied by a KCL academic, so Professor Ignac Fogelman was appointed. As he hadn't actually set papers before, I stayed on as Intercollegiate examiner until 2004.

The rubric for the course – now the MSc Nuclear Medicine – Science and Practice, GKTMS – read:

1. Entry Requirements
   • *A registrable qualification in Medicine awarded by UK university or a recognised European or overseas university.*
   • *Two years post-registration experience in general & acute medicine (to include management of medical emergencies*
   • *A mark of 6.5 in each section of IELTS examination or equivalent*

For limited GMC registration (*exemption from PLAB*):
- *As above but must pass at 7.0 in all sections of IELTS*

2. Curriculum

   The course consists of 6 modules of which 4 are taught. The 6 modules are:
   Physics & Basic Medical Science (*T*)
   Clinical & Diagnostic Nuclear Medicine (*T*)
   Radiopharmaceutical and Regulatory Aspects of Nuclear Medicine (*T*)
   Therapy, Radiation Protection & Radiobiology (*T*)
   Nuclear Medicine – Practical (*P*)
   Nuclear Medicine – Research (*R*)
   (*T = Taught, P = Practical and R = Research*)

3. Duration of programme of study
   Full-time: *1 year*
   Part-time: *2 years*

4. Examination
   Unseen written examinations: *2 Papers*
   End of Year 1 assessment viva (*part-time students*)
   Continuous assessment consisting of 5 Assessed essays of 2000 words each,
   logbook and 6 experiments
   Two oral examinations (*clinical and physics*)
   Dissertation/Report of 10,000 words and two Oral examinations.
   This may seem very organised, but an idea of the true state comes from an urgent
   fax sent to the students shortly before the exams:

Memo to students:
   Contrary to my previous memo there will be two written papers each of 3 h
duration.

   Paper 1 will have two parts.
   Part 1 – Radiopharmaceutical and Regulatory Aspects
   Part 2 -Physics and Basic Medical Science and
   It is recommended that students spend 1 h on Part 1 and 2 h on Part 2. Please
   bring a Scientific calculator to the examination.
   Paper 2 will have two parts.
   Part 1 – Therapy, Radiobiology and Radiation Protection
   Part 2 – Clinical/Diagnostic Nuclear Medicine
   It is recommended that students spend 1 h on Part 1 and 2 h on Part 2

There were five candidates, one of whom was unable to complete the examination as he had been called home for military service. It was possible to use the new flexibility of KCL and award him a diploma. There was a total of seven examiners!

This was also the last year of the University of London MSc – there was one candidate re-sitting from the previous year.

2000–2001 was the first proper year of the KCL course. There were eight students in the second year of taking the course part time, and six new students (two full-time and four part-time). There was a formal 70-page prospectus giving full details of the course.

In 2002–2003 there was a formal review by KCL, and the opportunity was taken to implement the options of having a Diploma and a Certificate.

A diploma course would still need a clinical attachment, but would not have a research module, whereas a certificate course would be a purely taught course with no practical or research and both should be able to use the MSc modules as they were.

Discussion took place concerning increasing the number of taught modules from 4 to 5. These modules would be examined in 4 papers as follows:

Paper 1: Physics & Basic Science
Paper 2: General Clinical (including GI, Neuro, Paediatric, Cardiovascular & Pulmonary Nuclear Medicine)
Paper 3: Radiopharmacy
Paper 4: Radiobiology & Radiation Protection and Therapy & Nuclear Medicine Oncology

This gave more flexibility for offering individual modules.

In 2005 came Modernising Medical Careers (MMC) and new training schemes.

There were hours of talks between RCP, RCR and BNMS about rationalising training schemes. There was also much heart-searching about what sort of specialty Nuclear Medicine was. One good outcome was that Nuclear Medicine was recognised as a shortage specialty. This led to the creation of several F2 (second-year) rotations with a Nuclear Medicine component.

In 2007–2008 there was the introduction of the concept of "Knowledge-Based Assessments" as an essential part of physician training. For some specialties it was a new exam – now known as a Specialty Certificate Examination.

For Nuclear Medicine, the Postgraduate Diploma was recognised. The MSc is recommended but not mandated and it was agreed in the 2007 and the 2010 Curriculum that the PG diploma was what was regarded as equivalent to the Specialty Certificate Examination of the other Physician specialties.

The MSc continues at King's College London https://www.kcl.ac.uk/prospectus/graduate/nuclear-medicine-science-and-practice, as part of a new training scheme designed to overcome the problems introduced by multimodality imaging including formal radiology training. However it's too soon to tell that story.

The current state of play is to be found at http://www.jrcptb.org.uk/specialties/nuclear-medicine.

References

1. Proceedings of the British Institute of Radiology. Br J Radiol. 1971;44(528):985–9.
2. Hilson AJW, Maisey MN, Brown CB, Ogg CS, Bewick MS. Dynamic renal transplant imaging with Tc-99m DTPA (Sn) supplemented by a transplant perfusion index in the management of renal transplants. J Nucl Med. 1978;19(9):994–1000.

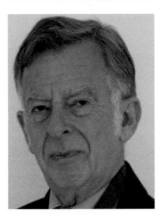

Andrew Hilson I qualified in 1967, when medicine was much simpler. My house jobs were in cardiothoracic surgery and medicine, and then I became SHO in intensive care (which didn't exist). Effectively I was an applied physiologist. As I wanted to be a general physician, I did further jobs in general medicine, neurology and rheumatology before being offered a locum position in endocrinology and nuclear medicine at Guy's hospital. I realised that this is what I wanted to do, and became Senior Registrar in Nuclear Medicine. This was a time of rapid growth – we bought the first 37-tube gamma camera in the UK, then the first LFOV camera, as well as one of the first dedicated computers – the DEC GAMMA-11 which had a full 16 k of memory. I developed an interest in renal nuclear medicine [2]. We moved from localising the placenta with a hand-held probe to using labelled RBCs, then gave it up when ultrasound came along. Phosphonate bone scanning revolutionised our work load, taking over from F-18-fluoride.

In 1983 I became a Consultant, half time at the Royal Free Hospital and half at the Institute of Urology. In 1993 the Institute moved into the Middlesex Hospital, and I became full- time at the Royal Free. Later Dr John Buscombe joined me.

The department had started in Medical Physics, where its specialism was pancreas imaging using a subtraction technique with Selenomethionine (taken up in the liver and pancreas) and Gold colloid (taken up only in the liver). It also had a long tradition of work with lung aerosols, so we carried out some of the early work on Technegas.

Because the Royal Free had a major liver unit, we were the first unit in the UK to use I-131-Lipiodol therapy for hepatocellular carcinoma. This led in turn to using In-111-Octreotide initially for diagnosis and then for therapy in neuro-endocrine tumours. The RFH now has a world-wide reputation in this field. We were leaders in scintimammography, which led to early involvement in sentinel node studies. This in turn led to my involvement in the "New Start" programme to teach sentinel node techniques to UK breast surgeons.

Inevitably, I became involved in medical politics. In addition to my involvement in the MSc, I was on the RCP Joint Specialty Committee from 2001, becoming Chair from 2004 to 2007; I served two terms on Council of the BNMS, becoming President from 2004 to 2006.

I have a strong interest in setting and improving standards, and was a member, of the National Audit and Standards Group (later Professional Standards and Education Committee) of the BNMS from 1995 to 2008 and was Chairman 2001–2004. I was a member of the Committee on Accreditation of Nuclear Medicine Departments, UEMS/EBNM) (2003–2014) and Vice-Chair 2010–2014. I was a member of the expert panel which led to the European Commission Radiation Protection report No 159 "European Commission Guidelines on Clinical Audit For Medical Radiological Practices (Diagnostic Radiology, Nuclear Medicine and Radiotherapy)".

I was an early member of the National Diagnostic Imaging Board and then was involved in the development of a national PET/CT strategy [2].

A Technologists Viewpoint

4

Liz Clarke

4.1   Training

In the early days training for technicians varied throughout the UK. In the 1980s in the Midlands for example there was a West Midlands Regional Health Authority training scheme in Medical Physics and Physiological Measurement. This 2 year course required "O" Level (GCSE) qualifications to include scientific subjects. It consisted of block release study for an Ordinary National Certificate (ONC) alongside hospital placements in Nuclear Medicine, Radiotherapy (Planning and Mould room), Radiation Protection, Audiology, Neurophysiology, Cardiology, and Renal units. Trainees then decided in which area they would like to specialise and could go on to pursue a Higher National Certificate (HNC) in this area. Again this could be a Regional training scheme or study in post.

The training of technologists has changed over the years to part time BSc course's with minimum requirement of "A" Level qualification which is run by a small number of universities. Additional modules allow for training on reporting, cardiac stressing and CT. This reflects the increased complexity of equipment and procedures now in place in departments and indeed the increased knowledge required to fulfil the role.

Specific courses were also developed to concentrate on the educational needs for radiographers in the use of radiopharmaceuticals in imaging. Radiography training was originally a 2 year diploma course and then progressed to a 3 year degree course. There is very little nuclear medicine training at undergraduate level and it has been necessary to continue to postgraduate training. Some staff have relied on in-house training with no formal qualification. Formal qualification originally was the Diploma in Nuclear Medicine of the College of Radiographers which came into existence around 1972,

L. Clarke
European Applications, GE Healthcare Ltd, The Grove Centre,
White Lion Road, Amersham HP7 9LL, UK

© The Author(s) 2016
R. McCready et al. (eds.), *A History of Radionuclide Studies in the UK:
50th Anniversary of the British Nuclear Medicine Society*,
DOI 10.1007/978-3-319-28624-2_4

prior to that it was a local course run by the Royal Marsden Hospital in Sutton. This included therapy and in-vitro work. This was phased out around 1983 by the College of Radiographers and replaced with the Diploma in Radionuclide Imaging (DRI) which was also open to technicians and was delivered in association with the Schools of Radiography. At present some universities organise Masters of Science degrees in nuclear medicine, with options to step off at post graduate diploma and post graduate certificate levels depending upon what level of education and training is needed.

The Register of Clinical Technologists (RCT) was established in 2000 with the aim of advocating statutory, professional regulation for Clinical Technologists (www.therct.org.uk). Clinical Physics Technologists are included on this register that includes: Scope of practice, Code of conduct and Continuing Professional Development. This register has recently received accreditation from the Professional Standards Authority and continues to strive for recognition as statutory regulation.

4.2   The Role

When radio-isotope departments were developed in the early 1950s most studies on patients involved laboratory based techniques using blood samples etc. Usually run by physicists who often made their own equipment with the investigations carried out by physics technicians.

As time and technology progressed, imaging became more important and while laboratory studies continued, physics technicians became more involved with patients. Early imaging was performed on a rectilinear scanner which produced very noisy images often on large paper prints. Things improved when single headed gamma cameras were introduced although achieving the correct exposure initially could be a problem. Large film cassettes were transported to communal dark rooms shared with Radiology to develop the films that were reliant on intensity and f-stop settings! Getting these wrong meant the repeat of an entire study. The advent of the Gamma Camera made life a lot easier. In Fig. 4.1 Neil Smith is imaging a patient with a Scintronix gamma camera in 1982. The images were still being recorded on x-ray film.

At this time although the jobs performed by both technicians and radiographers working in Nuclear Medicine departments were generally identical, working conditions such as weekly hours and annual leave entitlements were different. Today, following Agenda for Change, there is less difference between the two groups.

Cross sectional imaging started with SPECT and progressed to multimodality SPECT/ CT for attenuation correction, PET/CT and now PET/MRI. With the further introduction of multi-slice diagnostic CT scanners this itself raises the question of CT training for non-radiographers and also radiographers who have not had formal CT training. The introduction of University modules has helped to address this issue.

Every department will differ but generally the daily role has evolved to include radio pharmacy, dispensing, patient injection and supervision of cardiac stress sessions. The introduction of hybrid technologies has increased the complexity of acquiring and processing the studies leading to a demand for the staff to upskill. Some have undertaken further training to enable them to report and others are also business managers leading the technical side of their departments.

4.3   Research

Radiographers and technicians are often involved in strong research programs which have them taking a lead in the study itself; presenting and publishing the results. Dudley Road Hospital, Birmingham under the direction of Dr Keith Harding in particular led the way with its technicians presenting the results of their studies at the BNMS and International meetings, over 60 publications from their technologist team between 1985 and 2002 (Fig. 4.2). Topics covered a range of Nuclear Medicine procedures and Radiation Protection [1–4]. Nationally this practitioner involvement and enthusiasm has led to the introduction of dedicated Technologist sessions at

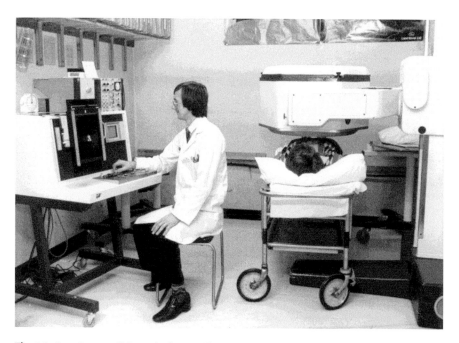

Fig. 4.1 Imaging on a Scintronix Gamma Camera in 1982

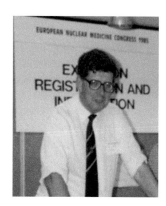

Fig. 4.2 Dr Keith Harding

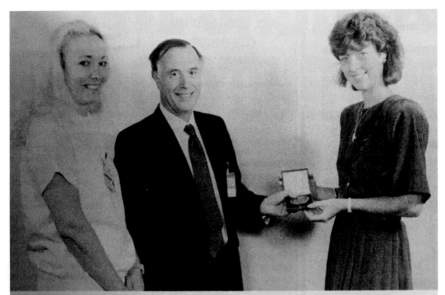

Pictured from left are Audrey Painter, Product Specialist (nuclear medicine) with Mallinckrodt Medical England, Dr Ralph McCready, chairman of the Task Group on Continuing Education, European Association of Nuclear Medicine, and prizewinner Liz Clarke.

Fig. 4.3 The first Mallinckrodt award for the best Technologist presentation at the EANM is presented to Liz Clarke (Courtesy Rad Magazine)

national and international meetings with proffered papers from across the UK and awards for best presentations. The first Mallinckrodt European Technologist award (META) for the best technologist presentation at the EANM was won by a UK technologist Liz Clarke (the senior technician at Dudley Road Hospital) Fig. 4.3 [5].

Another example of work by practitioners which in this case also included nurses was the publication of guidelines in Nuclear Medicine Communications for training for non-medical supervision of cardiac stress tests [6].

4.4   BNMS and Professional Development

At the EANM Congress 1989 in Strasbourg technicians and radiographers were refused entry into some clinical sessions. This led to an inaugural meeting of the first British Nuclear Medicine Society Technologist group which took place on the steps of the Congress centre. On their return to the UK the group began establishing itself in earnest with Caroline Townsend (Consultant Radiographer, UCH) as its first Chairperson and Liz Clarke as Secretary. A council consisting of a mix of technicians and radiographers from across UK and Ireland decided after much debate on the name of Technologists Group and a constitution was written. The group was

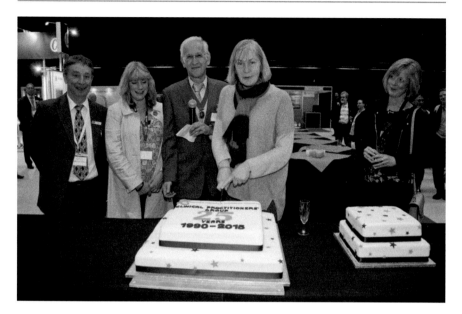

Fig. 4.4 The cake cutting ceremony at the celebration of the 25th anniversary of the BNMS clinical practitioner group. From left to right Ashby GB's Phil Facy, Mallinckrodt's Vicki Parkin, BNMS President Alp Notghi, Caroline Townsend (UCHL) and GE Healthcare's Liz Clarke (Courtesy Rad Magazine)

officially acknowledged as part of the BNMS in 1990. The EANM took our lead and established a European Technologist group established with the involvement of the UK a couple of years later. The aim of these groups was to unite all those working in all aspects of Nuclear Medicine regardless of their professional routes.

The name has recently changed again to Clinical Practitioners to better reflect the large variety and extent of expertise within the group. 2015 saw the celebration of 25 years of the group and a further change with the inclusion of nurses working within the specialty. It has been suggested that this may lead to a further change of name in 2016 (Fig. 4.4).

4.5 The Future

Radiographers and technologists continue to play a vital role in Nuclear Medicine.

They will have to ensure to increase their range of expertise to match the new technology and should embrace their opportunities to participate in research and continue their professional development.

Reporting of studies, research leading to PhDs, therapeutic administrations and Clinical Practitioner led patient clinics are just some of the extended advanced practice roles that are been undertaken.

References

1. Sherwin S, Donovan IA, Hesslewood SR, Sorgi M, Alexander-Williams J, Harding LK. Diethyl-HIDA concentration in bile, blood and urine. Nucl Med Commun. 1982;3:102 (Abstract).
2. Childs PO, Mostafa AB, Causer DA. A quantitative evaluation of breathing systems used with Kr-81m generators. J Nucl Med. 1983;24:157–9.
3. Allen C, De Bolla A, Tulley NJ, Harding LK, Barnes AD, Heath DA. The importance of the substraction technique in detecting parathyroid adenoma? Eur J Nucl Med. 1985;11:A47 (Abstract A251).
4. Clarke EA, Notghi A, Harding LK. Improving myocardial perfusion protocols: results of a UK survey. Nucl Med Commun. 2002;23:414 (Poster).
5. Clarke EA. Nuclear medicine: a safe occupation during pregnancy? Nucl Med Commun. 1989;10:260 (Abstract).
6. Jones I, Latus K, Bartle L, Gardner M, Parkin V. Clinical competence in myocardial perfusion scintigraphic stress testing: general guidelines and assessment. Nucl Med Commun. 2007; 28(7):575–82.

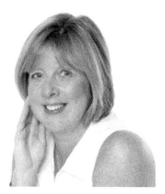

Liz Clarke European Applications Specialist Team Leader, GE Healthcare Life Sciences.

I worked in the Nuclear Medicine Department at Birmingham City Hospital (formerly Dudley Road) for 21 years. During that time I was involved in many research areas and presented many times at the BNMS and EANM. I was lucky enough to be awarded the Best Technologist paper on many occasions and was twice recipient of the Mallinckrodt award at the EANM. Much of this work was Radiation Protection orientated especially in regard to working during pregnancy and new imaging techniques in SLN imaging. Dr Keith Harding was my mentor whom I both feared and greatly respected simultaneously! I certainly owe all of my presenting skills to his superior knowledge and encouragement.

After great deliberation I left the NHS in 2002 to join Amersham Health (now GE Healthcare) to continue my career as an Applications Specialist. Although very different it has enabled me to further develop my expertise and continue to work within the Nuclear Medicine community, many of whom are now my friends as well as working colleagues.

Evolution of Nuclear Medicine Physics in the UK

5

Richard S. Lawson

Most nuclear medicine staff will know that the phenomenon of radioactivity was discovered by a Frenchman, Henri Becquerel [1]. However very few are aware that an Englishman nearly beat him to it. Silvanus Thompson was professor of physics at Finsbury Technical College in London and in 1896 he, like Becquerel, had been investigating the properties of certain phosphorescent minerals [2]. On 26th February he wrote to George Stokes, who was the President of The Royal Society, saying that he had discovered that uranium nitrate produced rays that penetrated paper and blackened a photographic plate. Stokes replied on 29th February advising him to publish without delay, but by 2nd March it was too late because on that day Becquerel presented his similar findings to the Academy of Sciences in Paris [2]. Nevertheless Sylvanus Thompson did make a contribution to medical imaging because in 1897 he became the first President of the Roentgen Society which later became the British Institute of Radiology [2].

Ernest Rutherford was born in New Zealand, but in 1895 he came to England to study in Cambridge under another Thompson, J.J. Thompson who discovered the electron. Here Rutherford identified two different components of the Becquerel radiation which he called alpha and beta rays [1]. In 1898 Rutherford took a post at McGill University in Montreal where, with Frederick Soddy, he investigated radioactive series and developed the disintegration theory of radioactivity [1]. However in 1907 he returned to the UK to take a position as Professor of Physics at Manchester University. Here, with Hans Geiger and Ernest Marsden, he performed the famous experiments on alpha particle scattering which led to him

R.S. Lawson
Department of Nuclear Medicine, Central Manchester Nuclear Medicine Centre, Manchester, UK

© The Author(s) 2016
R. McCready et al. (eds.), *A History of Radionuclide Studies in the UK:*
50th Anniversary of the British Nuclear Medicine Society,
DOI 10.1007/978-3-319-28624-2_5

proposing the nuclear theory of the atom. For this he was awarded the Nobel Prize in Chemistry in 1908 and in 1919 he became Professor of Physics in Cambridge [1]. For this work he is often known as the 'Father of Nuclear Physics'. Frederick Soddy returned to England to work at University College London where he and William Ramsay identified the alpha particle as a helium nucleus. In 1904 Soddy became a lecturer in physical chemistry at Glasgow University where he formulated the concept of isotopes of elements and for this he was awarded the Nobel Prize in Chemistry in 1921 [1].

One of Rutherford's students in Manchester in 1911 was a Hungarian chemist, George de Hevesy. Rutherford set him the task of trying to chemically separate the radioactive radium D from non-radioactive lead in pitchblende. His failure to do this led him to the conclusion that radium D must be an isotope of lead which would make an ideal tracer for stable lead [3]. De Hevesy is credited with the first ever use of a radioactive tracer when he added some radium D to the left-overs of a meal in his digs. When he was able to detect the radioactivity in the food that his landlady served up later in the week he was able to demonstrate that she was recycling old food rather than serving up fresh as she claimed [3]. De Hevesy subsequently went on to use his radioactive isotopes for more serious purposes as tracers in chemical reactions, in plants and then in animals [1]. For this work he received the Nobel Prize in Chemistry in 1943 and it is no wonder that he is known as the 'Father of Nuclear Medicine' [3].

In 1903 William Crookes, working in London, developed the first scintillation detector using zinc sulphide and this was used as the basis of scintillation detectors until it was superseded by sodium iodide some 40 years later [4]. However many early studies used a Geiger counter which was invented by Hans Geiger in Manchester in 1908 and later improved by Geiger and Walther Müller [4]. It is still used today as a versatile radiation detector.

The earliest nuclear medicine studies were performed without any imaging, just using blood or urine samples or external counting, initially with Geiger counters and later with scintillation detectors. One of the standard reference works for these studies was written by Norman Veall and Herbert Vetter in 1958 [5]. Norman Veall was a medical physicist at Hammersmith Hospital and then at Guy's Hospital who later became head of the Radioisotope Section at the MRC Clinical Research Centre at Northwick Park Hospital. He was talented at developing new equipment and pioneering its use for a wide variety of nuclear medicine studies. He developed the technique of measuring glomerular filtration rate using ^{51}Cr EDTA and pioneered techniques for thyroid function, blood flow, cardiac output and many others [6].

The first nuclear medicine study that produced anything like an 'image' of organ function was performed in Liverpool. In 1948 George Ansell and Joseph Rotblat used some of the first ^{131}I produced from the new reactor at Harwell to map the distribution of iodine uptake in a patient's thyroid [7]. For this they used a collimated Geiger counter that was manually positioned at different positions over the patient's neck. Like many other physicists Rotblat had worked on the Manhattan project during the war, but he quickly left the project on moral grounds and returned to his research in nuclear physics at Liverpool University. He became interested in the medical uses of radiation because he was determined that his work should be used for peace not war. In 1949 he became Professor of Physics at St Bartholomew's Hospital in London. In 1957, along with Bertrand Russell, Albert Einstein and others, he founded the Pugwash Conferences on Science and World Affairs, an organisation of scientists working for peace, and in 1995 he was awarded the Nobel Peace prize [1].

Automation of this mapping process led to development of the rectilinear scanner and the first British scanner was constructed in 1951 at the Royal Cancer Hospital in Sutton (now the Royal Marsden Hospital) by Val Mayneord. It could scan a Geiger counter repeatedly backwards and forwards over a small area building up a display on a cathode ray tube display [4]. In 1957 John Mallard at the Hammersmith Hospital produced a larger scanner with two scintillation detectors and a novel colour display [8]. This may have been the first whole-body clinical rectilinear scanner in Europe [9]. It was used for ^{131}I thyroid imaging and also for coincidence detection of positron emitting radionuclides in the brain [8, 9]. The existence of positrons and the phenomenon of positron-electron annihilation had been predicted by Paul Dirac whist working in Cambridge and he received the Nobel Prize for Physics in 1933 [1].

The first gamma camera in Europe was made by Ekco Electronics of Southend-on-Sea (formerly E.K. Cole Ltd). It improved on Anger's original design by having a storage oscilloscope display so that the image could be viewed in real time. The prototype was tested by John Mallard and Melvyn Myers at the Hammersmith Hospital in 1963 [9]. In 1965 John Mallard became Professor of Medical Physics at the University of Aberdeen and in 1967 they installed their first commercial gamma camera made by Nuclear Enterprises of Edinburgh [9]. In 1973 Mallard's Department developed the Aberdeen Section Scanner which was able to produce single tomographic slices of the brain from a pair of scintillation counters which scanned and then rotated around the patient's head [9]. In 1978 the Aberdeen department also developed a gamma camera SPECT system by mounting a Nuclear Enterprises gamma camera on a rotating gantry [9]. Nuclear Enterprises had started making gamma cameras after they purchased the nuclear instrumentation section of Ekco Electronics and subsequently Scintronix, another Edinburgh Company, continued development of a Scottish gamma camera. Figure 5.1 shows a Nuclear Enterprises gamma camera in use in Manchester Royal Infirmary about 1970.

Since the era of global equipment manufacturers, the opportunities for major developments in equipment by hospital physicists has largely disappeared. However, UK physicists have continued to play a vital role in developments and quality improvements in nuclear medicine procedures. Their contributions have often been as scientific and technical support to particular clinical problems, so it is more appropriate to mention them in the relevant clinical applications chapters of this book.

In 1994 the British Nuclear Medicine Society inaugurated a medal in memory of the pioneering work done by Norman Veall. The Norman Veall Medal is awarded

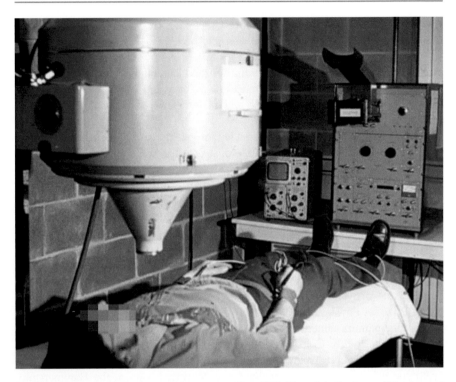

Fig. 5.1 A Nuclear Enterprises gamma camera circa 1970 (Copyright Institute of Physics and Engineering in Medicine 2013. Reproduced with permission)

annually to a clinical scientist who has made an outstanding contribution to the science and/or practice of nuclear medicine in the United Kingdom [10]. The list of recipients of the Norman Veall medal is therefore a good indication of some of the physicists and other scientists who have made important contributions to nuclear medicine in the UK in recent years. Recipients include Terry Jones and John Clark from the Hammersmith Hospital, John Mallard and Peter Sharpe from Aberdeen, Roger Ekins and Andrew Todd-Pokropek from University College Hospital, David Barber from Sheffield, John Fleming from Southampton, Alex Houston from Portsmouth, Peter Jarritt from Belfast, Malcolm Frier and Alan Perkins from Nottingham, Alex Elliott from Glasgow, David Williams from Sunderland, Robert Shields and Richard Lawson from Manchester, Steve Mather from Queen Mary University London, Glen Blake from Guy's and St Thomas' Hospital, Bill Thomson from Birmingham and Paul Maltby from Liverpool. These people have been involved in many different areas of nuclear medicine and their spread across the country shows that scientists continue to make important contributions to nuclear medicine throughout the UK.

References

1. L'Annunziata MF. Radioactivity: introduction and history. Amsterdam: Elsevier; 2007.
2. Thompson JS, Thompson HG. Silvanus Phillips Thompson, his life and letters. London: Fisher Unwin; 1920.
3. Myers WG. Georg Charles de Hevesy: the father of nuclear medicine. J Nucl Med. 1979;20(6):590–4.
4. McCready VR. Milestones in nuclear medicine. Eur J Nucl Med. 2000;27(Suppl):S49–79.
5. Veall N, Vetter H. Radioisotope techniques in clinical research and diagnosis. London: Butterworth & Co; 1958.
6. Maisey MN. Obituary, Dr Norman Veall. Nucl Med Commun. 1992;13:294.
7. Ansell G, Rotblat J. Radioactive iodine as a diagnostic aid for intrathoracic goitre. Br J Radiol. 1948;21:552–9.
8. Mallard J, Trott NG. Some aspects of the history of nuclear medicine in the United Kingdom. Semin Nucl Med. 1979;9:203–17.
9. Mallard JR. Hevesy memorial medal lecture 1985. Nucl Med Commun. 1987;8:691–710.
10. British Nuclear Medicine Society. The Norman Veal medal. http://www.bnms.org.uk/about/awards-prizes/the-norman-veall-medal.html. Last viewed 26 Oct 2015.

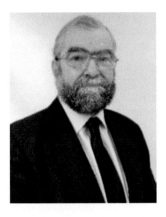

Richard S. Lawson Richard Lawson is now retired, but for 36 years he worked as a medical physicist in the Nuclear Medicine Department of Manchester Royal Infirmary which later became the Central Manchester Nuclear Medicine Centre. During that time he has taken a particular interest in renal studies and in teaching nuclear medicine. He was honoured to receive the Silver Medal of the Society and College of Radiographers for services to the teaching of radiographers and the Norman Veall Medal of the British Nuclear Medicine Society.

Nuclear medicine in Manchester Royal Infirmary started in 1967 when Tito Testa came over from Argentina bringing his skills as a nuclear medicine physician to conduct research for the Department of Surgical Gastroenterology. Initially radioisotope work was part of the Department of Medical Physics headed by Brian Pullan and in 1969 they moved into newly built facilities in a so-called 'Multi-purpose Building'. Robert Shields joined the hospital as medical physicist in 1971 and Nuclear Medicine became established as a Department in its own right, with Tito being appointed as its first consultant in 1974. Working together for over 30 years Tito and Robert have led a team of doctors, physicists, radiopharmacists and technologists who built up an international reputation for developing new nuclear medicine techniques, collaborating with clinical colleagues to introduce them into clinical practice. They have also always been involved with teaching and training nuclear medicine staff. In 1970 Tito's team developed pancreatic scanning techniques using ^{75}Se selenomethionine, first with a rectilinear scanner and later with a gamma camera and a computer subtraction technique to remove liver activity. In 1978 Paddy O'Reilly developed the technique of diuresis renography which is now used routinely throughout the world. The Department also pioneered the use of ^{123}I hippuran for gamma camera renography and promoted the use of nuclear medicine in monitoring kidney transplants. The team wrote a textbook on nuclear medicine in urology and nephrology and developed computer software for accurate analysis of renograms. The Department was an early investigator in the use of ^{99m}Tc HMPAO for brain perfusion imaging in dementia and an advocate of ventilation lung scans, with research on the use of ^{81m}Kr and ^{99m}Tc technegas led by Jackie James. More recently the Department has built up a reputation as a centre of excellence for nuclear cardiology led by Parthiban Arumugam and has introduced dose reduction techniques in several areas. Mary Prescott took over the reins of the Department from Tito when she became Clinical Director in 1999 and, together with Robert, introduced the PET service. In 2009 the Department finally moved out of the 40 year old Multi-purpose Building into brand new accommodation in the Central Manchester Nuclear Medicine Centre which incorporated a dedicated paediatric unit. In 2010 they became the only UK centre outside London to introduce a routine ^{82}Rb PET myocardial perfusion service, reducing both scan times and radiation dose for patients. Currently Parthiban Arumugam is the Clinical Director, Christine Tonge leads the physics team and Beverley Ellis heads the radiopharmacy.

The Institute of Nuclear Medicine London

6

Jamshed Bomanji and Peter J. Ell

Founded in 1961 with a first director (Professor J.E.Roberts 1961–1963), it developed under the direction of Professor E S Williams (1963–1985) and matured into international recognition under the director Professor Peter J. Ell (1986–2011). By its 50th anniversary, it already listed over 1000 peer reviewed publications, major Text Books and contributions to teaching. A significant milestone was achieved when the Editor of The Lancet commissioned the INM to edit 6 articles describing the clinical practice of Nuclear Medicine in subsequent 6 weekly issues of this premier medical publication (August 21 to September 25, 1999).

The physiological nature of the radionuclide tracer methodology is already transparent in the contents of the first 1961 INM Handbook for clinicians, highlighting the available procedures (Fig. 6.1). These included topographic surveys of the thyroid, liver, brain, haematological tests, such as red cell and platelet cell survival, plasma volume, vitamin B12 and iron absorption, iron clearance, as well as, inter alia, body composition studies with exchangeable sodium and potassium, extracellular fluid volume and total body water measurements. Thyroid function tests were part of the menu, including the assay of T4, the TSH stimulation test and perchlorate discharge testing.

J. Bomanji (✉)
Clinical Department, Institute of Nuclear Medicine, UCLH NHS Foundation Trust, 235 Euston Road, London NW1 2BU, UK

P.J. Ell
Department of Nuclear Medicine, Institute of Nuclear Medicine, UCLH NHS Foundation Trust, 235 Euston Road, London NW1 2BU, UK

© The Author(s) 2016
R. McCready et al. (eds.), *A History of Radionuclide Studies in the UK: 50th Anniversary of the British Nuclear Medicine Society*,
DOI 10.1007/978-3-319-28624-2_6

INSTITUTE OF
NUCLEAR MEDICINE
HANDBOOK

1st Edition, 1962

THE INSTITUTE OF NUCLEAR MEDICINE
THE MIDDLESEX HOSPITAL MEDICAL
SCHOOL
LONDON, W.1

MUSeum 8333. Extensions for Clinical Enquiries:
210 Clinical Tests; 243 Medical Officer

Fig. 6.1 1961 INM Handbook

Leading the speciality in the UK, the INM developed with the Royal Postgraduate Medical School and the Institute of Cancer Research, the first intercollegiate Master of Science Course (MSc) in Nuclear Medicine. This gained wide recognition, and at the INM, some 100 MSc graduates, mostly from overseas, obtained their diploma over the ensuing years.

The outstanding academic achievement has to be the development of radioimmunoassay and saturation analysis, under Professor Roger P. Ekins (deputy director 1968–1981), changing the world of analytical biochemistry, endocrinology and medicine. A Fellow of the Royal Society, Ekins received the Department of Health's Lifetime Achievement Award in 2011.

Other significant early contributions are highlighted below.

Edward Williams, as a life long mountaineer, investigated electrolyte function, aldosterone excretion and potassium retention at highest altitudes, publishing in Nature, inter alia, in 1961. A. Todd-Pokropek and D. Keeling designed and built in 1969 the first 3 D scanner in Europe, a true precursor of single photon emission tomography (SPET). The subsequent development of single photon emission tomography at the INM became a major success story, the Institute leading the UK in the clinical applications of the 3 D radionuclide imaging technology (with major peer reviewed output emerging from 1979 onwards).

The first UK patient studies with Gallium-67 citrate in 1970 in lymphoma by David Keeling and the development of deconvolution analysis in renography by Keith Britton and Nicholas Brown in 1968/1969, require to be highlighted here.

As novel radionuclide labelled tracers began to enable a transition to be made from mostly anatomical representation of organs (for example altered blood brain barrier imaging with pertechnetate, or liver imaging, even when mediated, for example, by Kupfer cell uptake) towards more pathophysiological meaningful pathway representations, the INM was able to keep at the forefront of what later would became known as molecular imaging. Hence the INM led the imaging with lypophilic tracers such as HMPAO for blood flow studies of the brain (1985), receptor imaging probes such as methoxybenzamide for imaging the D2/D3 dopaminergic system (1990), iomazenil for imaging the benzodiazepine receptor (1997), and investigating, inter alia, probes for the NMDA receptor (2003), for cell proliferation (2003), the 5-HT2A receptor (2006), the sigma-1 receptor (2006), and the somatostatin receptor in 2008.

A further first for the UK was the INM introduction of X-Ray based dual photon absorptiometry, in late 1988. This completely changed the accuracy and precision of bone mineral density measurements, the technology rapidly diffusing throughout the UK, with the newly established National Osteoporosis Society. In a short period of time, several seminal peer reviewed publications arose from the staff at the INM, such as in *BJR* 1989, *BJR* 1990, *EJNM* 1991.

By 1986, almost 25 % of all diagnostic procedures carried out at the INM involved the investigation of the heart (myocardial perfusion, wall motion, and ventricular ejection). The INM developed pharmacological stress testing with adenosine and dobutamine, with peer reviewed data in *BHJ* 1989, *JACC* and *AHJ* in 1991 and *Circulation* in 1998. Richard Underwood undertook a landmark study, with one the very few cost benefits studies published in the field of Nuclear Medicine (*European Heart Journal* 1999). A further first was the use of PETCT and Rb82, combining CT angiography with PET based perfusion, for myocardial studies (Groves 2007) followed by the introduction to the UK of solid state technology and dual radionuclide myocardial perfusion by Simona Ben Haim in 2010 (Fig. 6.2).

1972   **2010**   **1990**

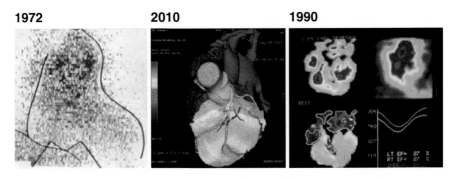

Fig. 6.2 Shows the evolving NM imaging technologies of the heart, from early K-42 studies in the 70s, to phase and amplitude with EF data in the 90s and Rb-52 PETCT in 2010

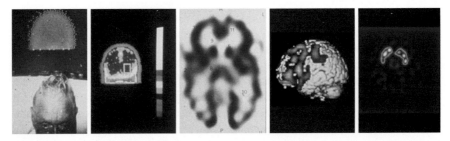

Fig. 6.3 Showing early BBB imaging, cerebral blood flow, MR co-registered benzodiazepine imaging and dopamine transporter imaging

From its early beginnings in the 60's and until the present time, the INM was always committed and involved in the development of imaging probes to study the brain, in its complexity and varied pathologies. Whilst a more detailed description is to be found in another chapter of this anniversary book, it is useful to recall the use of brain blood barrier scanning in the evaluation of patients with subdural haematoma, stroke, space occupying masses, the use of I123 and Tc99m labelled probes for the investigation of refractory temporal epilepsy, the dementias (Pick's and especially Alzheimer type) and the use of dopamine transporter probes for the investigation of essential tremor and Parkinsonian syndromes.(peer reviewed publications in, inter alia, *The Lancet* 1985, *Lancet* 1986, *Lancet* 1989, *BMJ* 1992, *Lancet* 1992 (Fig. 6.3).

From 1998 onwards, a major program in surgical oncology was developed at the INM It was based on a very simple but attractive concept, namely that lymph node progression in several major cancers is predictable and can be investigated when patients present with early disease. So the concept of the sentinel node and its biopsy was investigated in detail by the surgical and nuclear medicine teams (M. Keshtgar, W. Waddington, and P. Ell), with special emphasis of staging patients with early breast carcinoma. This novel technique proved to be extraordinarily effective, sparing invasive axillary surgery in 2 out of 3 patients presenting early with their condition. The INM started a major teaching program in the clinical skills lab, over 100 attendees benefited from their exposure to this training program, a Text Book and a CD was published and a substantial contribution to the literature ensued (inter alia, *Lancet* 1998, *Lancet* 1999, *Lancet Oncology* 2002, *J. National Cancer Institute* 2006, and *EJNM* 2000, *European J. Surgical Oncology* 2004).

6.1   UK Introduction of PETCT and PETMR

INM was first to introduce these major disruptive technologies to the UK (Ell PJ,von Schulthess GK. PET/CT: a new road map. *Eur J Nucl Med Mol Imaging*. Jun; 29(6):719–20, 2002) . The first UK patient to benefit from this new development was investigated with PETCT on the 17th of January 2002! PET/CT led to a dramatic increase in the acceptance and utility of the PET clinical programme – in the 3 months of September, October and November 2002, 402 patients were investigated with this unique technology. In a decade, over 100 peer reviewed INM publications were published (Fig. 6.4).

The management of patients with cancer changed, early staging and early treatment response have become paradigms of the clinical usefulness of this approach. As a multimodality imaging investigation, the referral base was rapidly extended to

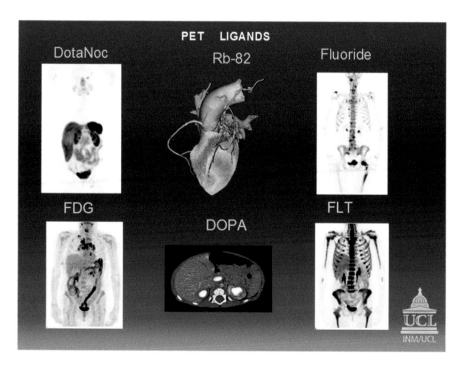

Fig. 6.4 Shows a range of labelled imaging probes which have been investigated at the INM with PETCT

include the assessment of cardiac function and coronary artery disease, and most recently, with PETMR, the early demonstration of amyloid plaque deposition in patients with cognitive impairment (early MID or developing AD). The Institute introduced PETMR to the UK in April 2012.

6.2 The Institute of Nuclear Medicine: National and International Impact on Standards, Teaching, Publishing and Organisation

Already mentioned above, the INM was a major contributer to an international recognised MSc course in Nuclear Medicine. Edward Williams, graduated in physics and medicine and became the first Chairman of ARSAC, the national body which issues medical certificates for safe practice. He was involved in writing much of the regulations which deliver safe radiation practice. Keshtgar, Waddington and Ell made a significant contribution to surgical standard setting for the practice of sentinel lymph node biopsy, now adopted by the Royal College of Surgeons as best practice. Peter Ell became Editor of the European Journal of Nuclear Medicine from 1988 to 2003, a major publication in the imaging field, raising the standard, profile and impact factor of this publication Keith Britton, whilst Consultant Physician in charge at INM, brought, as Congress President, the joint Congress of two European Societies of Nuclear Medicine to London in 1985. Britton and Ell wrote the new Bye Laws of the newly constituted single European Association of Nuclear Medicine, and were 2 of the 4 co-signatures founding the Association in 1985. Peter Ell became its President from 1994 to 1996. During his tenure, the European School of Nuclear Medicine was established.

Selected References

Ayres PJ, Hurter RC, Williams ES, Rundo J. Aldosterone excretion and potassium retention in subjects living at high altitude. Nature. 1961;191:78–80.
Cullum I, Ell PJ, Ryder J. X-Ray dual photon absorptiometry – a new method for the measurement of bone density. Br J Radiol. 1989;62:587–92.
Ekins RP. The estimation of thyroxine in human plasma by an electrophoretic technique. Clin Chimica Acta. 1960;5:453–9.
Ell PJ, Cullum I, Costa DC. Regional cerebral blood flow mapping with a new Tc-99m labelled compound. Lancet. 1985;II:50–1.

Groves AM, Speechly-Dick ME, Kayani I, Pugliese F, Endozo R, McEwan J, Menezes LJ, Habib SB, Prvulovich E, Ell PJ. First experience of combined cardiac PET/64-detector CT angiography with invasive angiographic validation. Eur J Nucl Med Mol Imaging. 2009;36(12):2027–33.

Gunning MG, Agnastopoulos C, Knight CJ, Ppper K, Burman ED, Davies G, Kox KM, Pennell DJ, ELL PJ, Underwood SR. Comparison of thallium-2o1, technetium-99m-tetrofosmin and dobutamine magnetic resonance imaging for identifying hibernating myocardium. Circulation. 1998;98(18):1869–74.

Keeling DH, Todd Pokropek AE. A new approach to brain scanning and Tomographic reconstruction. Proceedings of the second congress of the European Association of Radiology, Amsterdam. Amsterdam: Excerpta Medica; 1971

Keshgar M, ELL PJ. Sentinel lymph node biopsy in breast cancer. Lancet. 1998;352: 1471–2.

Sullivan R, Peppercorn J, Sikora K, Zalcberg J, Meropol NJ, Amir E, Khayat D, Boyle P, Autier P, Tannock IF, Fojo T, Siderov J, Williamson S, Camporesi S, McVie JG, Purushotham AD, Naredi P, Eggermont A, Brennan MF, Steinberg ML, De Ridder M, McCloskey SA, Verellen D, Roberts T, Storme G, Hicks RJ, Ell PJ, Hirsch BR, Carbone DP, Schulman KA, Catchpole P, Taylor D, Geissler J, Brinker NG, Meltzer D, Kerr D, Aapro M. Delivering affordable cancer care in high-income countries. Lancet Oncol. 2011;12(10):933–80.

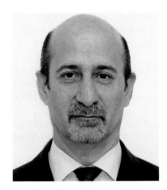

Dr. J Bomanji   Dr. J Bomanji completed his graduation in 1980. He did his post-graduation at St Bartholomew's Hospital where he completed his Masters and PhD in Nuclear Medicine in 1987. He was appointed as Consultant in Nuclear Medicine at St Bartholomew's Hospital in 1990 and then moved to The Middlesex Hospital in 1993, which is now part of the UCLH NHS Foundation Trust. Currently, he is the Clinical Lead and Head of Clinical Department at the Institute of Nuclear Medicine. His main interests are in the diagnostic and therapeutic application of nuclear medicine techniques in oncology, nephrology/urology, cardiology and neurology for benign and malignant disease.

He has contributed and published more than 200 research and clinical papers in peer-reviewed journals, authored numerous book chapters and is the editor of Nuclear Medicine in Oncology. He is assistant editor and advisory editor of various journals in the field of nuclear medicine.

A History of Nuclear Medicine in the UK Radionuclide Investigation of the Brain

7

Peter J. Ell

The composite figure below, best describes the development of radionuclide labelled probes at the Institute of Nuclear Medicine, and its commitment to investigating the brain, in health and disease. From the very early days of blood brain barrier imaging with labelled pertechnetate, and the use of 3″ and 5″ sodium iodide crystal scanners in the 60s, with added simple data processing in the 70s, progress was continuous, with the introduction of SPET, lyphophilic Tc99m labelled tracers for blood flow studies, investigating benzodiazepine receptor distribution in the female brain, the emergence of dopamine transporter imaging in patients with presumed Parkinson's disease, followed by PETCT and assessment of glucose metabolism with labelled FDG, and finally the UK introduction of PETMR and the investigation of the dementias, with labelled amyloid already in 2012 (Fig. 7.1).

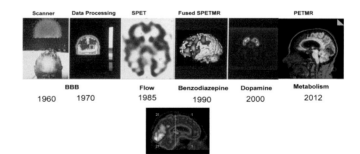

Fig. 7.1 Evolving Probes for Radionuclide Brain Imaging

P.J. Ell
Department of Nuclear Medicine, Institute of Nuclear Medicine,
University College London Hospitals,
UCLH NHS Foundation Trust, 235 Euston Road, London NW1 2BU, UK

© The Author(s) 2016
R. McCready et al. (eds.), *A History of Radionuclide Studies in the UK: 50th Anniversary of the British Nuclear Medicine Society*,
DOI 10.1007/978-3-319-28624-2_7

In 1985, scientists working at Amersham, UK, developed a first agent (hexamethylpropylenamine oxime –HMPAO – Ceretec) capable of traversing the intact blood brain barrier, with cerebral distribution according to blood flow (CBF). Capable of being labelled with Tc-99m, this discovery represented a major step in the development of imaging agents for single photon emission tomography. A first in man study was performed at the Institute of Nuclear Medicine and reported at a meeting of the British Institute of Radiology in February 1985.

This development, for which Amersham twice received Queen Industry Awards, led to a significant clinical program at the Institute. First patterns of regional cerebral blood flow were published (Lancet 1985), cerebral damage in HIV infection was studied (*Lancet* 1987), the patterns of CBF in dementia investigated (*J Cerebral Blood Flow and Metabolism* 1988 and *J. of Neurology, Neurosurgery and Psychiatry*, 1989). Patients with focal epilepsy were investigated (*Lancet* 1989 and *Neurology* 1992), stroke (*Lancet* 1989), follow up studies in dementia published (*JNM* 1989 and *J. Neurology, Neurosurgery and Psychiatry* 1991, *Brit. Med. J.* 1992), in traumatic intracerebral haematoma (*J. of Neurology, Neurosurgery and Psychiatry* 1991). A start in neuroactivation imaging was made (*European J Nuclear Medicine* 1991 and *J. of Neural Transmission* 1992), and the effect of depression on CBF investigated (J. of Affective disorders 1993).

This development led to one of the most productive research periods of the Institute, with a long list of peer reviewed publications. A clinical service was initiated, world wide HMPAO SPET is still the most common nuclear medicine imaging procedure for CBF studies.

The advent of PET would of course play a big role, even with the simple use of labelled glucose, a metabolic marker acting as a surrogate marker for brain blood flow, in most circumstances where the brain blood barrier is not impaired (such as epilepsy, and the dementias, for example). This has now led to a routine clinical activity in the investigation of non lesional patients with focal epilepsy (namely patients with normal or equivocal MR studies), where with FDG PETCT it is possible in one third of all referrals (in this difficult population) to offer clinical information with management utility.

7.1   Neuroreceptor Studies

With single photon emission tomography being at the time the only practical tomographic imaging technology for radiolabeled probes, Costa and staff at the Institute published very early on an important study, characterizing in vivo an I-123 labelled neuroreceptor for the D2/D3 dopaminergic system (*European J Nuclear Medicine* 1990) – 3-iodo-6-methoxybenzamide -IBZM. We show an IBZM study in a normal and a medicated patient, over a period of time, and the different degrees of receptor blockade in the striatum (Fig. 7.2).

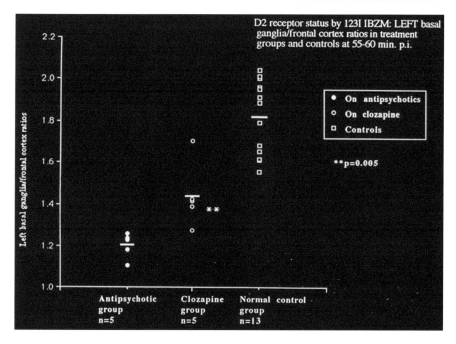

Fig. 7.2 Investigating the Clozapine Hypothesis

This was important work, and attracted to the Institute a young psychiatrist, from the Institute of Psychiatry at Denmark Hill (the late Lyn Pilowsky). Lyn was an enthusiastic researcher and soon obtained a Fellowship from the Medical Research Council (MRC).

Lyn was especially interested in managing patients with schizophrenia. There was indisputable pharmacological evidence for dopaminergic dysfunction in schizophrenia. Dopamine receptor blockade was shown to be an invariate requirement for the activity of antipsychotic drugs. The administration of clinical doses of antipsychotic medication resulted in a substantial degree of striatal D2 dopamine receptor occupancy in humans. Lyn wished to test the hypothesis that the D2 imaging ligand IBZM would be able to identify differences in D2 receptor activity in a population of schizophrenic patients (untreated drug naïve patients compared to controls, antipsychotic treated responders compared with non responders, and treated schizophrenic patients with tardive dyskinesia, compared with those without.

A seminal publication in The Lancet presented her findings : clozapine, single photon emission tomography, and the D2 dopamine blockade hypothesis of schizophrenia (*Lancet* 340, 199-202, 1992). The study showed beyond doubt that patients on typical antipsychotics showed poor response, despite D2 receptor blockade.

Significant clinical improvement occurred in all patients on clozapine, but at a lower level of D2 blockade by the drug. These findings suggested a more complex relation (rather than the hitherto suspected linear relation) between D2 blockade and clinical efficacy! In an important review in The Lancet, reviewing the 10 most important publications of that decade in psychiatry, Lyn's contribution was clearly acknowledged (Flaum and Andreasen 1997)

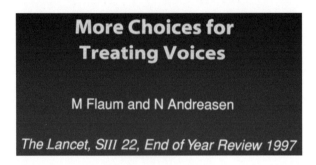

Between 1985 and 1990, some 40+ peer reviewed publications emanated from the Institute in respect to brain imaging. Whilst HMPAO became the most widely imaging probe used for blood flow SPET studies of the brain, other probes and approaches were investigated.

A further area of interest developed, with major input from the cardiac surgeons and psychologists. It was known for some time that patients undergoing coronary bypass surgery, often presented with a degree of cognitive impairment. If you were an excellent chess player pre-operatively, you may not be performing as well in the post operative period. To investigate organ function prior interventions, had met with recent success. One of our studies showed the clinical relevance of assessment cardiac ejection fraction prior aortic surgery. It was clearly possible to stratify patients into different risk categories (Mosley et al *Brit J Surgery* 1985, Ell *The Lancet* 1986).

And so it was decided to investigate brain blood flow, during and after 8 days and 8 weeks post coronary bypass surgery. Labelled xenon-133 was used for this purpose. A series of publications assessed the effect of surgery on this patients, the time required for their recovery and the modifications needed during surgery to minimise this risk (Smith et al., *the Lancet* 1986, Venn et al. *The Brit Heart J* 1987 and 1988, Treasure et al., *Europ J CardioTh Surgery* 1989).

Early studies with labelled HMPAO in patients with refractory and focal epilepsy showed the potential of interictal and ictal imaging. Again a number of publications emerged and a limited clinical service developed. In recent times a service has developed based on FDG PETCT and the investigation of MR non lesional patients with refractory and focal epilepsy. We show below a typical example where FDGPET aids in the localization of the epileptic focus (Fig. 7.3).

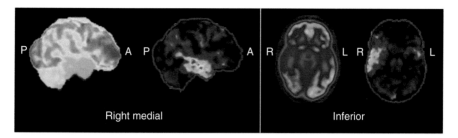

Right medial   Inferior

Fig. 7.3 Refractory epilepsy. Scalp video EEG telemetry suggests that focus arises from right frontal or temporal lobes. MRI is unremarkable. For intracranial EEG planning. There is focal right temporal lobe hypometabolism. Localization to right temporal lobe

Key References

Bressan RA, Erlandsson K, Jones HM, Mulligan R, Flanagan RJ, Ell PJ, Pilowsky LS. Is regionally selective D2/D3 dopamine occupancy sufficient for atypical antipsychotic effect? An in vivo quantitative [123I] epidepride SPET study of amisulpride-treated patients. Am J Psychiatr. 2003;160:1413–20.

Burns A, Philpot M, Costa DC, Ell PJ, Levy R. The investigation of Alzheimer's disease with single photon emission tomography. J Neurol Neurosurg Psychiatry. 1989;52:248–53.

Ell PJ, Jarritt PH, Deacon J, Brown NJG, Williams ES. Emission computerised tomography. A new diagnostic imaging technique. Lancet. 1978;II:608–10.

Ell PJ, Harrison M, Lui D. Cerebral blood flow with [123]Iodine labelled amines. Lancet. 1983;1:1348–52.

Ell PJ, Cullum I, Costa DC. Regional CBF mapping with a new Tc-99m labelled compound. Lancet. 1985;II:50–1.

Pilowsky LS, Costa DC, Ell PJ, Murray RM, Verhoeff NPLG, Kerwin RW. Clozapine, single photon emission tomography, and the D2 dopamine receptor blockade hypothesis in schizophrenia. Lancet. 1992;340:199–202.

Smith PLC, Newman SP, Ell PJ, Treasure T, Joseph P, Schneidau A, Harrison MJG. Cerebral consequences of cardiopulmonary bypass. Lancet. 1986;I:823–5.

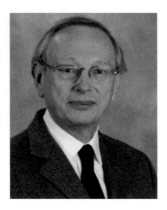

Peter J. Ell After graduation from Lisbon University in 1969, I became a junior staff member in a biology laboratory attached to a nuclear research reactor just outside Lisbon. My first assignment was to write a report for the Government, on the use of radiation as a method to sterilize once only use products, such as disposable syringes, then a true novelty. So I visited an establishment in Reading, produced my report, which led to a grant to attend the 2nd London University MSc degree course in nuclear medicine, in 1971. Many of us taped all the lectures, and we learned more about physics than nuclear medicine, and almost nothing about radiochemistry! I recall a comment from a colleague from Toronto, who, after hearing so many lectures on beta particles, enquired whether gamma rays where less relevant to nuclear medicine. After a 2 year stint as a Registrar at the INM and the Middlesex Hospital, I accepted a Lancet advertised post, to lead a new NM department in Feldkirch, Austria, in 1974. There I caused some local stir, for introducing radioim-munoassay's, in competition with a local conventional biochemistry lab, but obtained clear support from Vienna and the local Government.

1976 saw my appointment as Senior Lecturer at the Middlesex Hospital Medical School, not without trepidation and requesting a time off/cooling period, before acceptance (unheard off at the time). The CT scanner arrived at The Middlesex by end 1976 – by 1978, we published our first paper on single photon emission tomography. Cross sectional imaging and turf battles had truly arrived and changed our field. Progress and transformation was rapid, and it was fun! SPET became routine for most of our studies (brain, heart, lung, liver). Nuclear Medicine emerged as a separate medical speciality, recognized by the UEMS and Europe, through valiant effort from physicians working in Europe.

My appointment to the established UCL chair in Nuclear Medicine occurred in October 1987 – we had a great team of clinicians, physicists, pharmacists, nursing and technical staff, and plenty of post-graduates – again work was fun, fun breathes success, and success brings more fun. International commitments began to take place.

As first elected Secretary of the European Association of Nuclear Medicine (1987–1993), I was able to guide the development of this Society. With the European Industry Association for Nuclear Medicine, we discussed the future direction and regulatory practices of this medical speciality in Europe.

As the Editor in Chief of the European Journal of Nuclear Medicine (1990–2003), I was able to promote the science and medicine of nuclear medicine. The Impact Factor grew each year, beating the competition by the end of my term.

As the elected President of the European Association of Nuclear Medicine (1994–1996), I was responsible for the overall policy of the Association and its relationship with EC, UEMS, WHO, IAEA and WFNMB.

By January 2002, we introduced PETCT to the first UK patient – multimodality imaging was truly born. At my UCL retirement in 2009, and 38 years after arriving in London, PETMR was introduced to the INM and the UK.

Peter J. Ell FMedSci DR HC AΩA FRCP FRCR
Professor Emeritus UCL
Trustee University College London Hospitals Charity

A History of Nuclear Cardiology in the UK

8

S. Richard Underwood

8.1 Historical Perspective

The potential of radionuclides as tracers for the investigation of the circulation was realised many years ago but early experiments were hampered by primitive equipment. Blumgart and colleagues reported the first use of a radionuclide tracer in man in 1927. They used a cloud chamber to measure the transit time of intravenous radium C from one arm to the other and they noted much longer circulation times in patients with heart failure. In the late 1940s Prinzmetal and colleagues established the use of precordial time-activity curves following intravenous injection of a bolus of radionuclide. They used sodium-24 and a Geiger-Müller tube, but the technique was developed using iodine-131 and a more reliable scintillation counter by Shipley and colleagues, and was used by Huff and colleagues in conjunction with the Hamilton equation to measure cardiac output.

The first cardiac images were produced using a rectilinear scanner but further advances were made with the development of more suitable radioactive tracers and more sophisticated imaging equipment. In 1957 Anger's invention of the gamma camera opened the door for rapid development, initially with blood pool imaging, progressing to myocardial imaging, cardiac PET, and the multi-faceted discipline that is now an essential part of clinical cardiology (Table 8.1).

Along the way, UK-based researchers and clinicians have made significant contributions. Groups based in Aberdeen (cardiac PET), Northwick Park Hospital (technetium-based perfusion tracers), St Bartholomew's Hospital (first pass blood pool imaging), Hammersmith Hospital (cardiac PET), University College Hospitals

S.R. Underwood
Department of Nuclear Medicine, Imperial College London, Royal Brompton Hospital, Sydney St, London SW3 6NP, UK

© The Author(s) 2016
R. McCready et al. (eds.), *A History of Radionuclide Studies in the UK:*
50th Anniversary of the British Nuclear Medicine Society,
DOI 10.1007/978-3-319-28624-2_8

Table 8.1 Developing techniques in nuclear cardiology

Decade	Clinical developments
≤1960s	Experimental
1970s	Blood pool imaging
1980s	Thallium, diagnosis, cardiac cameras, pharmacological stress
1990s	Technetium perfusion tracers, prognosis, attenuation correction, reconstruction techniques
2000s	Hibernation, cost-effectiveness, solid state cameras, SPECT-CT, competing techniques
2010s	Patient outcome, new tracers, cardiac PET-CT, inflammation and infection imaging

(ECG-gated SPECT, rubidium-82, solid state cameras), Manchester Royal Infirmary (rubidium-82) and Royal Brompton & Harefield Hospitals (pharmacological stress, heart failure, cost-effectiveness) have all influenced the field internationally. The BNMS can be proud of the achievements of its members.

8.2   Radionuclide Ventriculography

In the late 1970s and early 1980s radionuclide ventriculography (RNV) was the main nuclear cardiology technique and it was used increasingly as an accurate and reproducible method of assessing left ventricular (LV) function. Although equilibrium imaging was most commonly used, first pass imaging had particular advantages for assessing right ventricular function and intra-cardiac shunting, as successfully used by the paediatric cardiologists at Guy's Hospital [1]. Parametric imaging provided simple methods of visualising regional function from the phase and amplitude images [2]. The Institute of Nuclear Medicine under the guidance of Peter Ell at the Middlesex Hospital demonstrated the value of such functional imaging in clinical practice (Fig. 8.1), and the phase image in particular continues to be of interest in assessing ventricular dysynchrony before resynchronisation pacing in patients with heart failure. This group also pioneered gated blood pool tomography [3] but with only two 100 ms frames per cardiac cycle it was not until image acquisition and processing techniques improved that it became a realistic technique as used today.

The simplicity and reproducibility of RNV meant that it was the technique of choice for serial assessments of LV function in patients having cardiotoxic chemotherapy or after heart transplantation but the increasing availability of echocardiography and its lack of ionising radiation led to it effectively replacing RNV. The availability of accurate methods of assessing LV function from gated myocardial SPECT led to a further decline, although RNV remains a valuable technique when echocardiography or magnetic resonance imaging (MRI) are not possible.

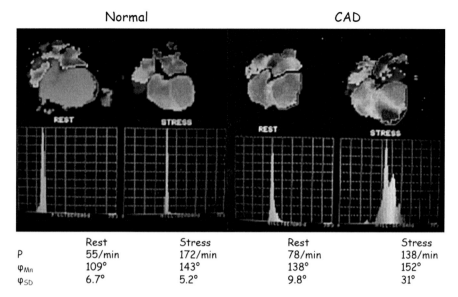

	Rest	Stress	Rest	Stress
P	55/min	172/min	78/min	138/min
φ_{Mn}	109°	143°	138°	152°
φ_{SD}	6.7°	5.2°	9.8°	31°

Fig. 8.1 The phase image and LV phase histograms from equilibrium radionuclide ventriculography acquired at rest and during maximal dynamic exercise in a patient without coronary disease (*left*) and one with significant left anterior descending disease (*right*). Mean phase (φ_{Mn}) increases with heart rate (*P*) but the standard deviation of phase (φ_{SD}) broadens in the patient with LAD disease indicating delayed contraction in the relevant area. The standard deviation of the phase histogram is a sensitive method of detecting inducible ischaemia

8.3   Myocardial Perfusion Scintigraphy

As RNV was becoming less popular, so the combined assessment of myocardial viability and perfusion using thallium-201 and technetium-99m MIBI and tetrofosmin developed. Myocardial perfusion scintigraphy (MPS) is now the dominant nuclear cardiology technique that should be available to all cardiac services although appropriate expertise is not always available and there are still UK sites that rely on other techniques for coronary functional imaging. Planar MPS was effectively replaced by SPECT in the 1980s and it has developed from a diagnostic technique to a method of assessing prognosis and hence guiding clinical management and improving clinical outcome in patients with coronary artery disease (CAD). MPS SPECT has also become an alternative to FDG PET in assessing patients with ischaemic LV dysfunction and possible hibernating myocardium (Fig. 8.2) [4].

When the technetium-99m labelled perfusion tracers, MIBI and tetrofosmin were introduced in the 1990s many sites switched entirely to these despite some of their disadvantages [5]. Apart from commercial marketing, one driver for the change was the lower radiation burden of the technetium tracers. However, several recalculations

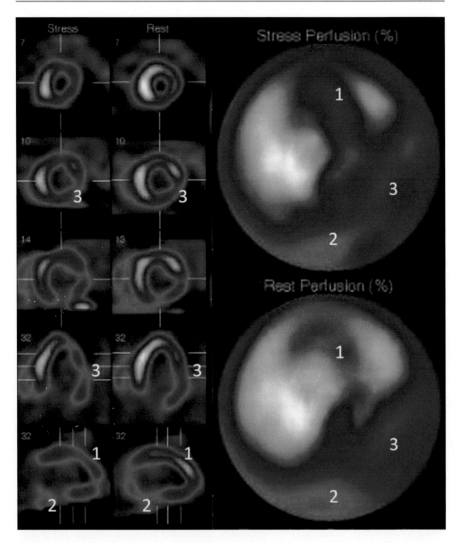

Fig. 8.2 Myocardial perfusion scintigraphy in an patient with ischaemic heart disease and heart failure. The antero-apical region (*1*) is almost fully viable but has inducible hypoperfusion. ECG-gating showed it also to be akinetic without thickening and hence hibernating. There is also transmural infarction of the basal inferior wall (*2*) extending as partial thickness scarring of the infero-lateral region (*3*). LVEF was 30 % but improved to 48 % after revascularisation

have almost equalised the effective doses at 6, 7 and 8 mSv for 1000 MBq of tetrofosmin, MIBI and 80 MBq of thallium respectively [6]. With this new information and the superior uptake characteristics for the quantification of perfusion in absolute terms using dynamic SPECT, thallium MPS may yet see a resurgence.

8.4   Pharmacological stress

One of the strengths of MPS is that it is not necessary for the patient to exercise maximally and pharmacological stress of myocardial perfusion became particularly prevalent in the UK in the 1980s and beyond, such that it is now used in the majority of studies instead of dynamic exercise. The coronary vasodilator dipyridamole was initially used following validation work by Gould in dogs and it is still the commonest pharmacological stressor in countries such as France, primarily because it is cheap. The Royal Brompton group was among the first to combine it with dynamic exercise in order to improve image quality and reduce side effects [7]. They later extended this to adenosine stress [8], which effectively replaced dipyridamole in the UK because of its shorter half-life and hence safety and practicality. They were also the first group in Europe to use the more specific A2a adenosine receptor agonist, regadenoson [9], which extended the options for stressing patients with obstructive airways disease and potentially also those with conducting tissue disease.

8.5   NICE and the UK Societies

As the NICE programme of clinical guidelines and technology appraisals grew in the 1990s it was apparent that the focus of healthcare providers was moving from evidence of effectiveness to cost-effectiveness to clinical outcomes. At this stage there were only computer-based estimates of cost effectiveness with no supporting clinical studies. However, in 1999 clinical cost-effectiveness studies from the UK [10] and USA [11] provided strong support for MPS at a time when there was no similar evidence to support alternatives. The data were considered by NICE and formed part of the evidence for the first technology appraisal of an imaging technique in cardiology [12]. More recently, the Cambridge group led what is still the only prospective randomised study of non-invasive imaging compared with invasive angiography and confirmed the cost-effectiveness of MPS compared with echocardiography and MRI [13].

In assisting the technology appraisal of MPS, the BNMS, BNCS and other professional bodies collaborated to review the evidence for MPS in clinical practice and the resulting publication became the most quoted EJNM publication in 2008 [14]. Since then, an alphabet cocktail of studies (BARI, COURAGE, DEFER, ERASE, FAME, GRACE, INSPIRE, etc.) has shown, among other things, that ischaemia-guided intervention in patients with CAD leads to better clinical outcomes. It should now be unusual for patients with stable disease to undergo revascularisation procedures without some form of functional assessment. The challenge for the future will be to show the advantages of doing this by nuclear cardiology in preference to alternative techniques that in some centres have replaced nuclear cardiology because of more ready access to expertise and equipment.

8.6   The Future

Whether nuclear cardiology will move towards PET from SPECT is unclear. FDG PET is already very valuable for the assessment of myocardial inflammation and infection, such as in sarcoidosis and infected devices (Fig. 8.3).

For perfusion imaging the future is less clear. UK groups have been at the fore-front of using rubidium-82 PET, the only perfusion technique that is feasible with-out an on-site cyclotron, but PET may not gain wide acceptance until more cost-effective techniques become available, possibly such as flurpiridaz, a fluorine-18 labelled perfusion tracer currently in phase 3 trials. In addition, the availability of high resolution and sensitive solid state cameras with the ability to quantify per-fusion may challenge PET (Fig. 8.4) [15, 16].

There is the prospect of moving nuclear cardiology into the world of electro-physiology interventions, such as ablation of atrial fibrillation and ventricular arrhythmias. Pilot studies between University College and Royal Brompton Hospitals and have shown that mIBG combined with a solid state camera can local-ise ganglionated plexi of the sympathetic nervous system that are related to the control of arrhythmia and are potential targets for intervention (Fig. 8.5).

Reports of the demise of nuclear cardiology have therefore been exaggerated. Its future seems assured provided that we continue our proud history within the BNMS of contributing to research, education and clinical application in the field.

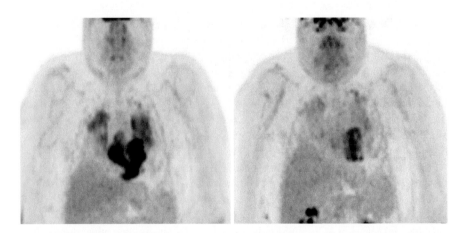

Fig. 8.3 FDG PET in the coronal plane in a patient with cardiac sarcoidosis before (*left*) and 10 months after steroid therapy (*right*). The images are acquired in the fasting state to suppress normal myocardial glucose metabolism. There is intense abnormal activity in the heart and hilar regions that is partially suppressed after treatment (Courtesy Dr K Wechalekar, Royal Brompton Hospital)

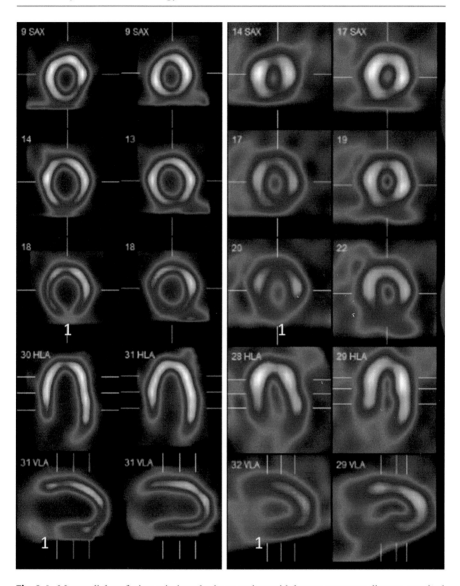

Fig. 8.4 Myocardial perfusion scintigraphy in an patient with known coronary disease, acquired using a solid state gamma camera in 4 min (*left*) and a conventional camera in 12 min (*right*). In each case stress tomograms are on the left and rest on the right. Both studies show an inducible perfusion abnormality of the basal inferior wall (*1*) but the superior spatial and contrast resolution of the solid state camera is obvious

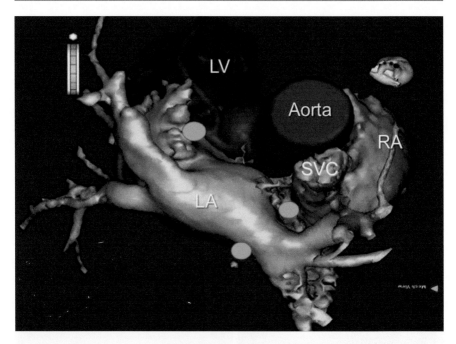

Fig. 8.5 Segmented CT scan with the sites of ganglionated plexi (GPs) superimposed (*green ovals*) imaged using iodine-123 mIBG and a solid state gamma camera. The fused images can be imported into the electrophysiology laboratory system to aid localisation of the GPs and ablation (Courtesy Dr Sabine Ernst, Royal Brompton Hospital). *LA* left atrium, *LV* left ventricle, *RA* right atrium, *SVC* superior vena cava

References

1. Baker EJ, Ellam SV, Lorber A, Jones OD, Tynan MJ, Maisey MN. Superiority of radionuclide over oximetric measurement of left to right shunts. Br Heart J. 1985;53:535–40.
2. Underwood SR, Walton S, Laming PJ, Ell PJ, Emanuel RW, Swanton RH. Quantitative phase analysis in the assessment of coronary artery disease. Br Heart J. 1989;61:14–22.
3. Underwood SR, Walton S, Ell PJ, Jarritt PH, Emanuel RW, Swanton RH. Gated blood pool emission tomography: a new technique for the investigation of cardiac structure and function. Eur J Nucl Med. 1985;10:332–7.

4. Gunning MG, Anagnostopoulos C, Knight CJ, Pepper JR, Burman ED, Davies G, Fox KM, Pennell DJ, Ell PJ, Underwood SR. Comparison of Tl-201, technetium-99m tetrofosmin and dobutamine magnetic resonance imaging in identifying hibernating myocardium. Circulation. 1998;98:1869–74.
5. Kapur A, Latus KA, Davies G, Dhawan R, Eastick S, Jarritt PH, Roussakis G, Young M, Anagnostopoulos C, Bomanji J, Costa D, Pennell DJ, Prvulovich EM, Ell PJ, Underwood SR. A comparison of three radionuclide myocardial perfusion tracers in clinical practice: the ROBUST study. Eur J Nucl Med Mol Imaging. 2002;29:1608–16.
6. Andersson M, Johansson L, Minarik D, Leide-Svegborn S, Mattsson S. Effective dose to adult patients from 338 radiopharmaceuticals estimated using ICRP biokinetic data, ICRP/ICRU computational reference phantoms and ICRP 2007 tissue weighting factors. Eur J Nucl Med Mol Imaging Phys. 2014;1:9.
7. Pennell DJ, Mavrogeni S, Anagnostopoulos C, Ell PJ, Underwood SR. Thallium myocardial perfusion tomography using intravenous dipyridamole combined with maximal dynamic exercise. Nucl Med Commun. 1993;14:939–45.
8. Pennell DJ, Mavrogeni S, Forbat SM, Karwatowski SP, Underwood SR. Adenosine combined with dynamic exercise for myocardial perfusion imaging. J Am Coll Cardiol. 1995;25: 1300–9.
9. Brinkert M, Reyes E, Walker S, Latus KA, Maenhout AF, Mizumoto R, Nkomo Q, Standbridge K, Wechalekar K, Underwood SR. Regadenoson in Europe: first-year experience of regadenoson stress combined with submaximal exercise in patients undergoing myocardial perfusion scintigraphy. Eur J Nucl Med Mol Imaging. 2014;41:511–21.
10. Underwood SR, Godman B, Salyani S, Ogle J, Ell PJ. Economics of myocardial perfusion imaging in Europe: the EMPIRE study. Eur Heart J. 1999;20:157–66.
11. Shaw LJ, Hachamovitch R, Berman DS, Marwick TH, Lauer MS, Heller GV, Iskandrian AE, Kesler KL, Travin MI, Lewin HC, Hendel RC, Borges-Neto S, Miller DD. The economic consequences of available diagnostic and prognostic strategies for the evaluation of stable angina patients: an observational assessment of the value of precatheterisation ischaemia. J Am Coll Cardiol. 1999;33:661–9.
12. NICE technology appraisal guidance [TA73]. Myocardial perfusion scintigraphy for the diagnosis and management of angina and myocardial infarction. https://www.nice.org.uk/guidance/ta73. Accessed 8 Nov 2015.
13. Thom H, West NEJ, Hughes V, Dyer M, Buxton M, Sharples LD, Jackson CH, Crean AM, Armstrong J, Buxton M, Caine N, Coulden R, Crean A, Dyer M, Gillham M, Goddard H, Goldsmith K, Hughes V, Lee E, Patel R, Schofield P, Sharples L, Sonnex E, Stone D, Treacy C. Cost-effectiveness of initial stress cardiovascular MR, stress SPECT or stress echocardiography as a gate-keeper test, compared with upfront invasive coronary angiography in the investigation and management of patients with stable chest pain: mid-term outcomes from the CECaT randomised controlled trial. BMJ Open. 2014;4:e003419.
14. Underwood SR, Anagnostopoulos C, Cerqueria MD, Ell PJ, Flint E, Harbinson MT, Kelion A, Al-Mohammad A, Prvulovich EM, Shaw LJ, Tweddel AC. Myocardial perfusion scintigraphy: the evidence. Eur J Nucl Med. 2004;31:261–91.
15. Ben-Haim S, Murthy VL, Breault C, Allie R, Sitek A, Roth N, Fantony J, Moore SC, Park M-A, Kijewski M, Haroon A, Slomka P, Erlandsson K, Baavour R, Zilberstien Y, Bomanji J, Carli MFD. Quantification of myocardial perfusion reserve using dynamic SPECT imaging in humans: a feasibility study. J Nucl Med. 2013;54:873–9.
16. Chowdhury FU, Vaidyanathan S, Bould M, Marsh J, Trickett C, Dodds K, Clark TPR, Sapsford RJ, Dickinson CJ, Patel CN, Thorley PJ. Rapid-acquisition myocardial perfusion scintigraphy (MPS) on a novel gamma camera using multipinhole collimation and miniaturized cadmium–zinc–telluride (CZT) detectors: prognostic value and diagnostic accuracy in a 'real-world' nuclear cardiology service. Eur Heart J Cardiovasc Imaging. 2014;15:275–83.

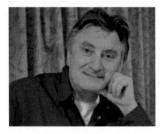

S. Richard Underwood   Richard Underwood gained a first class honours degree in chemistry at Merton College, University of Oxford, which included a period working in George Radda's laboratory using NMR and ESR in biological systems. He went on to study medicine, graduating in 1977. After general medical training he specialised in cardiac medicine learning both noninvasive and invasive techniques, and for the last 20 years he has practised noninvasive cardiac imaging, with major clinical and research interests in nuclear cardiology, magnetic resonance and in cardiovascular X-ray computed tomography.

Since 1985, Professor Underwood has worked at Royal Brompton Hospital, London and its academic wing, the National Heart and Lung Institute, Imperial College School of Medicine. He has been closely involved in the development of magnetic resonance techniques for the investigation of the cardiovascular system, and has contributed substantially to its progression from research technique to every-day clinical tool. His current research interests include the assessment of myocardial perfusion using pharmacological stress, the characterisation of hibernating myocardium, and the cost-effectiveness of cardiac imaging techniques. He has published and lectured widely and has directed or co-directed important training courses on nuclear cardiology at national and international level.

He is professor of cardiac imaging at the National Heart and Lung Institute, Imperial College London, and honorary consultant at Royal Brompton & Harefield Hospitals. External commitments include past-chairman of the ESC working group on nuclear cardiology and magnetic resonance, past-chair of the British Nuclear Cardiology Society and the International Congress of Nuclear Cardiology, and current member of the European Council on Nuclear Cardiology.

Non-medical interests include aviation, skiing and gastronomy.

S Richard Underwood, DM, FRCP, FRCR

Professor of Cardiac Imaging, Imperial College London

Great Ormond Street Hospital for Children, Paediatric Nuclear Medicine in the UK

9

Lorenzo Biassoni

The history of paediatric nuclear medicine in the United Kingdom is closely related to Great Ormond Street Hospital (GOSH) for Children. The hospital was founded in 1852 and is one of the most famous children's hospitals in the world, a centre of excellence which gathers expertise and equipment to treat complex paediatric clinical conditions.

Paediatric nuclear medicine at GOSH is inseparably linked to Professor Isky Gordon (Fig. 9.1), who was a consultant radiologist with special interest in nuclear medicine at GOSH between 1976 and 2006 and the clinical lead of the nuclear medicine unit within the radiology department.

The first Gamma Camera was installed at GOSH in 1977. This was a Nuclear Enterprises camera with a hard copy real time output. It took a further 4 years before a dedicated computer, Informatek, was purchased. The pediatricians found the

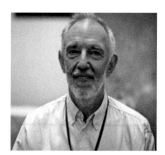

Fig. 9.1 Prof. Isky Gordon

L. Biassoni
Department of Radiology, Great Ormond Street Hospital for Children NHS Foundation Trust, London WC1N 3JH, UK

© The Author(s) 2016
R. McCready et al. (eds.), *A History of Radionuclide Studies in the UK: 50th Anniversary of the British Nuclear Medicine Society*,
DOI 10.1007/978-3-319-28624-2_9

functional information on patho-physiology from nuclear medicine examinations useful, although there was a significant period of training for both radiologists and paediatricians. Quite quickly renal nuclear medicine examinations began replacing conventional radiology, something that the older paediatricians did not readily accept. Soon nuclear medicine examinations were being used in most areas of the body. The nuclear medicine expanded at GOSH so that by 1995, there were three gamma cameras, including one mobile unit. Exciting research came from close working with different groups of paediatricians both at GOSH and at Institute of Child Health (UCL ICH).

Within the European Association of Nuclear Medicine (EANM), as it is known today, Dr Amy Piepsz from Brussels and Isky Gordon from London met in Barcelona in 1978 and decided that a special group interested in paediatric nuclear medicine should be created. Over the next few years, with a few 'political' skirmishes the task group in paediatrics was formed in the EANM, with contributions also from several other colleagues among whom Klaus Hahn from Munich, Rune Sixt from Gothenburg, and Isabel Roca from Barcelona. GOSH played a leading role in the task group, the group produced two atlases of bone scintigraphy in children, created guidelines for virtually every paediatric nuclear medicine examination and generated research that resulted in published papers.

The Henri Becquerel fellowship was established at GOSH. The fellowship was aimed at nuclear medicine physicians from the developing world who had at least 4 years experience in nuclear medicine to come to GOSH for 6 months. The cost was fully funded by the nuclear medicine section of the department of radiology. Thirteen Henri Becquerel fellowship were awarded to nuclear medicine physicians from 12 countries.

Professor Gordon has been an international figure and brought the paediatric nuclear medicine activity of GOSH to the world stage. Under his leadership the nuclear medicine unit of GOSH have set the standards of quality of paediatric nuclear medicine examinations in the UK and abroad. The unit developed its own philosophy and practice in preparing the child and family for the examination and became also a reference point to train radiographers and technicians. The child is not a small adult and paediatric nuclear medicine is like a suit made to measure for each child: among other innovations, the unit designed and adopted a novel system of image acquisition, with a custom made cut out gamma camera acquisition table, still in use today in a new version (Fig. 9.2): the table has a hole in the middle of the same size of the gamma camera head, so that the child lies directly on the collimator, thus significantly improving the resolution of the images.

Gordon did ground breaking work in the use of nuclear medicine techniques in nephro-urology. He developed the concept that slow drainage in dynamic renography in the context of an ante-natally diagnosed hydronephrosis, does not necessarily mean obstruction. Together with his physicist Peter Anderson he set up a new cutting edge way to process the renogram: the clearance image, a purely functional image that reflects renal parenchymal function per pixel (very much loved by the surgeons, who used to call it "the poor man's DMSA"), the pelvic excretion

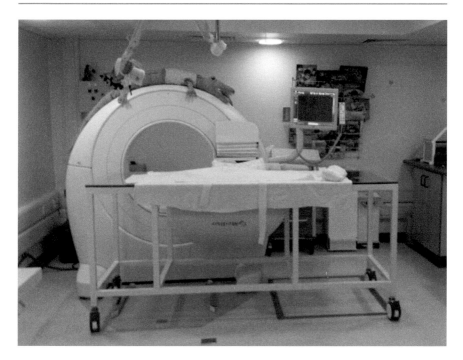

Fig. 9.2 Custom made cut out gamma camera acquisition table

efficiency (PEE), an index to evaluate drainage taking renal function into account, the post-micturition view normalized to the dynamic renography, which takes into account gravity in the evaluation of drainage. Gordon developed the indirect radionuclide cystography (IRC) as a way to make the best possible use of the information available at the end of the renogram to evaluate the possible presence of vesico-ureteric reflux and to gain some insights on bladder function. He disseminated around the world all his findings in countless invited lectures at national and international conferences, and crystalized his practice in the European and British Guidelines on paediatric renography, of which he was a main contributor.

The Nuclear Medicine Unit at GOSH pioneered radionuclide studies on intractable epilepsy. The technique for paediatric ictal and interictal cerebral perfusion studies in children with epilepsy in the UK was set up at GOSH. Over the years, several other paediatric nuclear medicine centres in the UK established links with GOSH to get advice. GOSH was also to take a leading role in the molecular imaging assessment of children with neuroblastoma. The SIOPEN High Risk Neuroblastoma Study Group received a significant contribution from the nuclear medicine unit at GOSH with the MIBG studies. The quality of the GOSH MIBG studies was acknowledged to be outstanding in Europe, their number per annum among the highest. Professor Gordon authored the first Guidelines of the European Association of Nuclear Medicine (EANM) on MIBG scintigraphy in children in 2002.

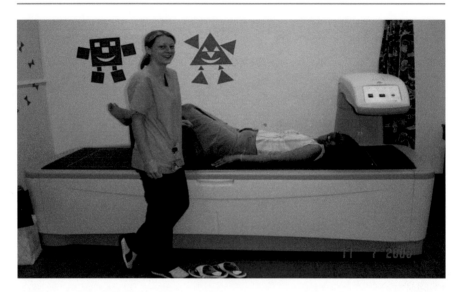

Fig. 9.3 Bone densitometry scanner

In the year 2000 a bone densitometry scanner was purchased (Fig. 9.3), as well as a third gamma camera, as part of the expansion of the Nuclear Medicine Unit. With the help of the now Professor Mary Fewtrell, a paediatrician of the Nutrition Unit in the Institute of Child Health, a correction for the height and weight of the child was introduced, thus enabling a proper evaluation of the bone density results in children.

In 2008 the Nuclear Medicine Unit moved to a different part of the hospital, in a new purpose built more spacious department. A new Siemens Symbia T2 SPECT CT gamma camera was installed (Fig. 9.4). In the following year, child friendly low dose CT acquisition protocols were developed, with the help of senior CT radiographers. With these protocols, the CT component of the examination is SPECT guided and limited to the area of clinical interest, and administers a very low radiation dose, often below 0.5 mSv. Gradually a new area of expansion of the clinical service was opening up, with a significantly increase in referrals for bone scans with SPECT CT in children and adolescents with back pain and extremity pain, in requests for DMSA with SPECT CT in children with renal stones, and of MIBG scans with SPECT CT in neuroblastoma patients.

By the end of 2015, more than 400 SPECT CT examinations have been performed in children and adolescents, and preliminary results on the effectiveness of SPECT CT in paediatrics in different pathologies have been presented at national and international conferences. This is an expanding activity of the department, linked to the recent upgrade of the Hermes workstations that allows accurate co-registration of tomographic nuclear medicine images with CT and/or MRI performed separately.

In the last 3 years there has been a significant increase of the activity of the nuclear medicine unit in the field of gastrointestinal motility studies, thus meeting a long standing request from the Gastroenterology Department. The unit has made

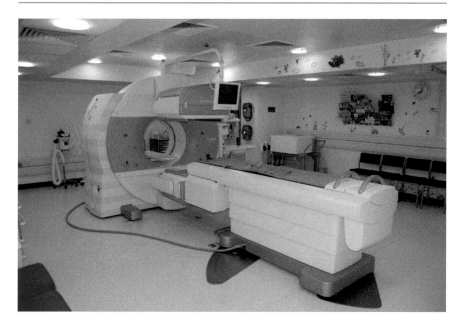

Fig. 9.4   Siemens Symbia T2 SPECT CT gamma camera

available studies for the evaluation of colonic and small bowel transit in children with severe constipation, thus helping significantly clinical management.

Visitors to the department have continued to come from different parts of the world, especially the Indian subcontinent, and are allowing the establishment of professional links with those countries.

In recent years, the nuclear medicine unit has been involved in a project funded by the International Atomic Energy Agency (IAEA), geared to publishing a book on everyday practice of paediatric nuclear medicine. This publication will disseminate, especially in developing countries, part of the vast practical experience accumulated at GOSH over many years.

In conclusion, the paediatric nuclear medicine unit at GOSH has been and still is a reference point of paediatric nuclear medicine practice in the UK and abroad. Ground breaking work has been done and novel work is in progress for the better management of many children affected by a broad spectrum of pathologies.

Key References

Gordon I, Colarinha P, Fettich J, Fischer S, Frokjaer J, Hahn K, Kabasakal L, Mitjavila M, Olivier P, Piepsz A, Porn U, van Velzen J. Guidelines for standard and diuretic renography in children. www.eanm.org/Publications/Guidelines

Gordon I. Assessment of paediatric hydronephrosis using output efficiency. J Nucl Med. 1997;38:1487–9.

Anderson PJ, Rangarajan V, Gordon I. Assessment of drainage in PUJ dilatation: pelvic excretion efficiency as an index of renal function. Nucl Med Commun. 1997;18:826–9.

Gordon I, Mialdea Fernandez RM, Peters AM. Pelvic-ureteric junction obstruction. The value of post-micturition view in 99m-Tc-DTPA renography. Br J Urol. 1988;61:409–12.

Moorthy I, Easty M, McHugh K, Rideout D, Biassoni L, Gordon I. The presence of vesicoureteric reflux does not identify a population at risk for renal scarring following a first urinary tract infection. Arch Dis Child. 2005;90:733–6.

Hahn K, Fischer S, Gordon I. Atlas of bone scintigraphy in the developing paediatric skeleton. Berlin/Heidelberg: Springer; 1993. ISBN 978-3-642-84945-9.

Gordon I, Fischer S, Hahn K. Atlas of bone scintigraphy in the pathological paediatric skeleton. Berlin/New York: Springer; 1996. ISBN 978-3-642-61060-8.

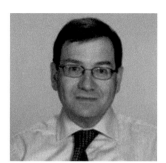

Lorenzo Biassoni I graduated in Medicine from the University of Rome "La Sapienza" and I undertook a specialty residency programme in Oncology at the University of Genoa. During this time I was fascinated by the developing use of nuclear medicine in Oncology, also stimulated by the example of my father, who was a general physician and university professor with special interest in thyroid diseases and in nuclear medicine. As a result, I decided to pursue a career in Nuclear Medicine. I enrolled in the specialist training programme in Nuclear Medicine at the University of Genoa. Subsequently I undertook the Master Degree programme in Nuclear Medicine at the University of London, while based at St Bartholomew's Hospital under Professor Keith Britton. I continued my training in Nuclear Medicine in London at Guy's Hospital under Professor Michael Maisey. After a number of locum jobs in different London hospitals, in 1999 I was appointed consultant in nuclear medicine at Barking, Havering and Redbridge NHS Trust, where I worked as a single handed consultant for almost 3 years. I subsequently joined Great Ormond Street Hospital for Children in 2002 (where I had worked before) and I had the chance to work closely with Professor Isky Gordon for almost 5 years. In 2006, following Professor Gordon's retirement from the NHS, I succeeded him as Clinical Lead of the Nuclear Medicine Unit at GOSH. I also work for Barts Health NHS Trust 1 day a week, gaining experience in PET CT imaging. During my time at GOSH I have been involved in the Paediatric Committee of the EANM, which I chaired between 2004 and 2007. I also joined the Nuclear Medicine Committee of the British Institute of Radiology (BIR), where I served for 7 years. In 2007 I joined ARSAC as a paediatric nuclear medicine expert, and I served on that Committee for 8 years. In 2008 I was elected Fellow of the Royal College of Physicians. I am on the editorial board of the *European Journal of Nuclear Medicine and Molecular Imaging*, of *Molecular Imaging & Radiometabolic Therapy*, and of the *Journal of Cancer and Allied Specialties*, and the Associate Editor for Nuclear Medicine of the *BJR Case Reports*. I am a reviewer for several other scientific journals. I am passionate about teaching and I have organized many regional, national and international teaching events on paediatric nuclear medicine. I have been invited to give many lectures at national and international conferences. Currently my main goal is to expand the range of the examinations on offer at the Nuclear Medicine Department at GOSH. My research interests include nuclear medicine in paediatric oncology and nephro-urology, and SPECT CT in paediatrics. I have authored 35 papers in peer-reviewed journals and 8 chapters of textbooks.

Keith Britton

Our adventure with the kidneys started at the then Middlesex Hospital culminating in 1971 with Britton and Brown's monograph Clinical Renography [1]. This was prefaced: 'The disciplines of Medicine and Physics are like oil and vinegar – often shaken together, often appetising but not easily miscible'. We attempted to 'blend the soothing oil of medicine with the acid reality of Physics in a study of common interest: how the kidney works'. We debunked the old nomenclature of the reno-gram – the Vascular spike, the Secretory phase and the Excretory phase – for exam-ple the latter is the 'left behind in the kidney' phase. We proposed 'Second phase' for the rising portion and 'Third phase' for the descending portion of the renal activ-ity time curve. We cleaned up the renogram with Computer assisted blood back-ground subtracted, CABBS, Renography [2]. With a grant from the Leverhulme Trust, we developed a mobile Renography trolley and couch with Nuclear Enterprises of Edinburgh, which could be taken to the Intensive care unit and the patient transferred onto it.

NJG, Nick, Brown first showed the importance of the integral of the Blood clear-ance curve [1, 3], later used as the Patlak or Rutland plot (Mike Rutland did his MSc with us). It led to the numerical approach to measuring the Outflow Efficiency. Nick also developed various renal transit times.

K. Britton
Departments of Radiology and Nuclear Medicine, The London Clinic,
20 Devonshire Place, London W1G 6BW, UK

© The Author(s) 2016
R. McCready et al. (eds.), *A History of Radionuclide Studies in the UK:*
50th Anniversary of the British Nuclear Medicine Society,
DOI 10.1007/978-3-319-28624-2_10

10.1   Essential Hypertension

Using the bimodal distribution of transit times, we were able to separate the contributions of the Cortical and Juxta-medullary nephrons to renal blood flow [4]. These were validated in animal studies with Steve Wilkinson at King's College. We were able to show that in Essential Hypertension, Cortical blood flow is reduced and Medullary blood flow is increased [5], the former increasing salt retention and the latter accounting for loss of urine concentrating ability, Nocturia being a common symptom of early Hypertension. We were also able to show that Captopril greatly improved Cortical nephron flow and reduced blood pressure. It led to Lancet publications of the hypothesis 'Renin and Renal Autoregulation' [6] and 'Essential Hypertension: a disorder of cortical nephron control' [7].

10.2   Measurement Based Medicine

These approaches were based on the premise that numerical indices of renal radionuclide studies were better than eye-balling and guessing the meaning of a complex activity time curve. Indeed our philosophy became a wish to substitute 'Evidence based medicine' which applied to the many with 'Measurement based medicine' which applied to the individual through 'Normal ranges' and 'Action determining ranges'. For example in adults one should act to save a kidney with more than 15 % of total renal function, but not if it is less that 5 % of total. Sreenevasan's dictum was made during my IAEA time in Malaysia 'In the presence of bilateral outflow obstruction (usually uric acid stones) always operate on the kidney with the better relative function first as determined by renography' [8].

The refinements occurred at St Bartholomew's Hospital in the City of London through the Physicist Cyril Nimmon's expertise and dedication. The Gamma camera replaced the probes and his advanced computer programmes enhanced and simplified the results [9].

10.3   Outflow Efficiency

The Outflow efficiency [10] is determined by subtracting the renal activity time curve from the integral of the blood clearance curve (the input curve) fitted to its second phase to give the integral of the output curve. This output curve is then taken as a percentage of the input curve. Unlike Frusemide dependent measurements, it is independent of the level of renal function. Normally a kidney should excrete over 78 % of what it took up within 30 min.

10.4   Transit Times

Renal Transit times seem to confuse some practitioners. Think of 'Pooh sticks'. On one side of the bridge a bunch of sticks are thrown into the stream together. You run to the other side of the bridge and see one stick coming out first followed by a distribution of others. The distribution of times they take to pass under the bridge can be measured and a mean time of transit determined. The mathematical process is Deconvolution. The result tends to be noisy. Three factors made it usable. Firstly the high count rate given by Tc-99m MAG3. This was first used in the UK in our department and published by Dr now Professor Adil Al Nahhas [11]. Secondly Cyril Nimmon devised two constraints on the activity time curve, monotonicity and non-negativity; and a lack of over-smoothing of the original data; thirdly the use of the left ventricle to give the blood clearance curve as a high count input.

The understanding of Transit times by the clinician may be likened to learning to ride a bicycle. One falls off several times at the start and either gives up as many have; or persists until one avoids the potholes and is rewarded by the ride.

10.5   Renovascular Disorders

It may be noted that renal radionuclide studies do not generally distinguish between large and small vessel renal disease if they are functionally significant in contributing to hypertension. The Mean Parenchymal Transit Time, MPTT is normally less than 240 s. In the context of Hypertension due to Renovascular disorder such as Renal artery stenosis, it exceeds this and indicates the narrowing is functionally significant. It is further increased in this context by Captopril, particularly in large vessel disease. Gruenewald et al. [12], who did his MSc with us, showed that if MPTT was prolonged then most hypertensive patients are benefitted by revascularisation or stenting with a reduction of their Blood Pressure, but if MPTT was normal in this context, none of the Hypertensive patients benefitted.

10.6   Obstructing Uropathy

Consider some basics, there is the Force from cardiac output, which does not change if there is a stone blocking urine flow. There is the Resistance to urine flow. The consequence of the interaction of a Force and a Resistance is a rise in Pressure. Pressure is not a cause but a consequence. Pressure is equal and opposite in all directions (Sir Isaac Newton) so there is no such thing as 'back pressure'. When there is a system of fluid in a tube, it flows from the higher pressure to the lower pressure. A non reabsorbable agent such as Tc-99m MAG3 therefore takes time to travel down this pressure gradient. In Obstructing Uropathy, the resistance to flow increased so the solute takes longer to transit. Increased resistance to flow is thus transmutable into an increased transit time which can be measured. In this context the Parenchymal Transit Time Index, PTTI is helpful. It is measured as the MPTT minus the Minimum (shortest) Transit time which makes an allowance for different urine flow rates. Normal PTTI is less than 156 s. Unlike Frusemide based studies, it is independent on the level of renal function, although there has to be sufficient function for the measurement to be made. The Urologist Mr Hugh Whitfield at St Barts gained the Hunterian award for evaluating the advantages of using PTTI in the context of potential Obstructing Uropathy [13, 14]. An abnormal PTTI is one of the earliest indicators of functionally significant Obstructing Uropathy in adults, for example when renal function is still normal. It is also independent of the size of the renal pelvis. If the words 'outflow obstruction' or worse 'partial obstruction' were replaced by 'increased resistance to flow', the understanding of an 'outflow obstruction' would be made easier.

The above is a simplification of Transit time usage, which needs some interpretive skill, for example PTTI may be unreliable if MPTT is abnormal. Transit time indices should be taken together with other clinical information and renal measurements in a holistic approach.

10.7   Frusemide Response

There are a number of ways of evaluating the response to Frusemide. Visually one may compare the rising second phase with the falling third phase of the activity time curve. If the rate of fall of the third phase before or after Frusemide is appropriate to the rate of rise of the second phase, then no Obstructive Nephopathy is likely. However using a T1/2 or other measure of the rate of fall of the third phase will be normal if renal function is good and abnormal if renal function is poor. It is not to be relied upon. Our usual protocol is to inject Frusemide at 16 min (F + 16) so that one can see the visual effect of Frusemide on any pelvic retention of tracer and its effect on the third phase of the activity time curve. When Frusemide is given 15 min before the start of the renal activity time curve, (F-15), which was previously used when the renogram was equivocal, the response to Frusemide cannot be assessed, except by comparison with a previous study without F-15. F-15 often causes the patient urinary urgency and may cause early termination of the study.

The numerical indices Outflow efficiency [15] and Parenchymal transit time index [16] avoid the need for F-15 in equivocal studies.

Whereas MAG3 is anionically bound, Cyclosporine is cationically bound in the kidney, hence the lack of reliability of Tc-99mMAG3 in this context of renal transplantation. Ajit Padhy and Kishor Solanki developed a new cationic binding agent Tc-99m DACH intended for the evaluation of cyclosporine toxicity [17]. Jamshed Bomanji among many other contributions showed the early beneficial effects of Lithotripsy on the outcome of the treatment of renal calculi [18]. We developed a 'bootstrap' model of the 'Counter Current' mechanism of urinary concentration with our systems analysis colleagues from City University [19]. In conclusion we emphasised that Nuclear Medicine allowed the appreciation and measurement of renal physiology and patho-physiological processes in man.

Since this section was to be related mainly to the work at St Bartholomew's Hospital, I apologize for being unable to mention the works of many others in renal function measurements, renal transplants, renal tumours and Paediatrics. With their help, Renal Radionuclide studies have an established place in Nephrology and Urology.

References

1. Britton KE, Brown NJG. Clinical renography. London: Lloyd Luke; 1971.
2. Britton KE, Brown NJG. Computer Assisted Blood Background Subtraction (CABBS) renography in obstructive nephropathy. Proc Roy Soc Med. 1970;63:1246–7.
3. Brown NJG, Britton KE. The renogram and its quantitation. Br J Urol. 1969;41(Suppl):15–25.
4. Britton KE. The measurement of intrarenal blood flow distribution in man. Clin Sci Mol Med. 1979;56:101–4.
5. Gruenewald SM, Nimmon CC, Nawaz MK, Britton KE. A non-invasive gamma camera technique for the measurement of intrarenal flow distribution in man. Clin Sci (London). 1981;61:385–9.
6. Britton KE. Renin and renal autoregulation. Lancet. 1968;2:329–33.
7. Britton KE. Essential hypertension: a disorder of cortical nephron control? Lancet. 1981;ii:900–2.
8. Sreenevasan G. Bilateral renal calculi. Ann Roy Coll Surg Engl. 1974;55:3–12.
9. Britton KE, Brown NJG, Nimmon CC. Clinical renography: 25 years on. Eur J Nucl Med. 1996;23:1541–6.
10. Chaiwatanarat T, Padhy AK, Bomanji JB, et al. Validation of renal output efficiency as an objective quantitative parameter in the evaluation of upper urinary tract obstruction. J Nucl Med. 1993;34:845–8.
11. Al Nahhas AA, Jafri RA, Britton KE, et al. Clinical experience with 99mTc-MAG3 mercaptoacetyl triglycine and a comparison with 99mTc-DTPA. Eur J Nucl Med. 1988;14:453–62.
12. Greuenewald SM, Stewart JH, Simmons KC, Crocker EF. Predictive value of quantitative renography for successful treatment of atherosclerotic renovascular hypertension. Aust N Z J Med. 1985;15:617–22.
13. Whitfield HN, Britton KE, Nimmon CC, Hendry WF, Wallace DM, Wickham JE. Renal transit time measurements in the diagnosis of ureteric obstruction. Br J Urol. 1981;53:500–3.
14. Britton KE, Nimmon CC, Whitfield HN, et al. Obstructive nephropathy, successful evaluation with radionuclides. Lancet. 1979;1:905–7.
15. Cosgriff PS, Morrish O. The value of output efficiency measurement in resolving equivocal Frusemide responses. Nucl Med Commun. 2000;21:390–1.
16. Britton KE, Nawaz MK, Whitfield HN, et al. Obstructive nephropathy: comparison between Parenchymal transit time index and Frusemide diuresis. Br J Urol. 1987;59:127–32.
17. Padhy AK, Solanki KK, Bomanji J, et al. Clinical evaluation of Tc-99m Diamino-cyclohexane, a renal agent with cationic transport: results in healthy normal volunteers. Nephron. 1993;65:294–8.
18. Bomanji J, Boddy SAM, Britton KE, et al. Radionuclide evaluation of pre- and post-extracorporeal shock wave lithotripsy for renal calculi. J Nucl Med. 1987;28:1284–9.
19. Britton KE, Cage PE, Carson ER. A 'bootstrap' model of the renal medulla. Postgrad Med J. 1976;52:279–84.

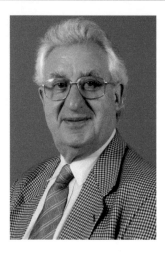

Keith Britton I was educated at Malvern College, Downing College, Cambridge and the then Middlesex Hospital, London. I was registrar to Dr John Nabarro and Dr 'Willy' Slater and carried out the hospital's first renal dialysis. I became fascinated with Nuclear Medicine as a non-invasive tool to study how organs functioned in people and not just their anatomy. I studied with Prof Edward Williams at the Institute of Nuclear Medicine, Middlesex Hospital gaining the MSc; and an MD at Cambridge examined by Professor Norman Veall. He said that he had repeated my work on renal transit times and agreed with it. That was the exam! I became registrar to Professor Stanley Peart at St Mary's Hospital, learning about the management of Hypertension. This prepared me for my part in the Hypertension Clinic at St Bartholomew's Hospital. I was appointed as a General Physician at St Barts. If the clinic staff could not decide on the specialty to which a GP had referred a patient, then it would go to me as a generalist to sort out in the outpatient clinic.

I then became a Professor of Nuclear Medicine at the Medical school and Queen Mary College, giving up my ward duties at St Barts. I was made director of the Nuclear Medicine group of Cancer Research UK, which funded staff and equipment to carry out research into imaging and therapy with radio-labelled monoclonal antibodies in cancers. During my time and work with the International Atomic Energy Agency, we were able to welcome over 100 overseas postgraduate doctors to sit the MSc in Nuclear Medicine, most passed. As a past President of the Society of Nuclear Medicine, Europe, I was able to help to found the European Association of Nuclear Medicine, EANM and lead the congress in 1985 at the Barbican centre in London.

I was a past President of the BNMS and organised that Physicists became full members. I was one of the founder editors of Nuclear Medicine Communications and of the World Journal of Nuclear Medicine. I published over 250 peer reviewed manuscripts and several books including Clinical Nuclear Medicine, lead Editor Professor Michael Maisey, going on for four editions.

After my retirement due to age 65, I was awarded Emeritus Professor, University of London. I became Chair of the Board of the independent Cromwell Hospital for two and a half years. It was revealing to be able to manage instead of being managed by the NHS. I continue in private practice as Consultant in Nuclear Medicine to The London Clinic and the London Bridge Hospital.

St Bartholomew's Hospital and Medical School: Department of Nuclear Medicine

11

Keith Britton

11.1 Personal Reflections

It was started by the Nobel prize-winning Professor Sir Joseph Rotblatt in 1960 as a Radioisotope department with Ms McAlister and Mr Laurie Hawkins as Physicists. I was appointed by the Chief of Radiology Dr Ian Kelsy-Fry as Consultant Physician in charge of the Nuclear Medicine Department in 1976. My aim was to set up an open, friendly and welcoming clinical, teaching and research department in spite of the poor physical environment and initially only one gamma camera. It was mainly equipped through various grants including one from the St Barts Trustees and not by the NHS. I was also appointed as Consultant Physician in acute General Medicine with ward beds, 'on take' twice a week, Outpatients and Hypertension Clinic and with students to teach. After I was made Professor of Nuclear Medicine, I continued with the Hypertension Clinic but with no further ward duties. We had excellent Physicist support with Messrs Alex Elliot, Cyril Nimmon, Melvyn Carroll, Ravin Sobnack and for therapy Ms Ro Foley; and innovative Pharmacy support with Mr Stephen Mather and Mr Kishor Solanki and their staff. Mr Jagdish Mistry led the dedicated technical staff with Ms Nishamalie Fenando. We introduced and were the first to use the Hermes system in the UK.

The three main influences that helped determine the teaching, research and staffing were the International Atomic Energy Agency, IAEA, the Imperial Cancer Research Fund, ICRF, later renamed Cancer Research UK and the European Association of Nuclear Medicine, EANM.

K. Britton
Departments of Radiology and Nuclear Medicine, The London Clinic,
20 Devonshire Place, London W1G 6BW, UK

© The Author(s) 2016
R. McCready et al. (eds.), *A History of Radionuclide Studies in the UK:*
50th Anniversary of the British Nuclear Medicine Society,
DOI 10.1007/978-3-319-28624-2_11

11.2 IAEA

For 25 years, I undertook between one to three annual mainly teaching missions abroad for the IAEA in many different countries. As a result and with their support over 100 post-graduate doctors from overseas came to us. They undertook and almost all passed the MSc of the University of London. They are mostly now Heads of Nuclear Medicine departments around the world, for example Drs Mike Rutland in New Zealand, Simon Gruenewald in Australia, Vaseem Chengazi in USA, Husein Kartamihardja in Indonesia, Ng Chensiew in Malaysia, Kerim Sonmezoglu in Turkey and Mirek Dzuik in Poland; and in the UK, included Dr Jamshed Bomanji, who was our longest and most active resident, Dr now Professor Sobhan Vinjamuri, Dr Hikmat Jan and Dr Lorenzo Biassoni. Several British residents and many other short and longer term visitors including Dr now Professor Adil Al Nahhas joined us. Commonwealth scholars also made their mark including Professor Ajit Padhy who became Head of Life Sciences at the IAEA. There were 9 PhDs doctorates on different aspects of the department's research. Among other innovative work, Kishor Solanki and I developed Infection imaging with Tc-99m Ciprofloxacin 'Infecton'. Ciprofloxacin binds specifically to dividing bacteria including Mycobacteria. It was patented through the government's British Technology Group, BTG (now a stock market quoted company). The IAEA supported a multi-centre study in eight countries from Indonesia to Argentina. Over 1000 patients were recruited. The results were excellent and published by the IAEA and elsewhere. Infecton was taken over by the Canadian company DraxImage. Kishor Solanki subsequently joined the IAEA.

11.3 IRCF

Dr Marie Granowska joined the department in 1976 supported by the Wellcome Foundation to develop non-invasive measurement of Cerebral Blood flow in ml/min using Tc-99m Albumin or Red Cells with Cyril Nimmon's computer programmes. She showed that Cerebral Blood flow improved in Professor John Lumley's patients with carotid artery disease after extra-cranial intra-cranial bypass surgery.

The ICRF supported her to undertake clinical research using the monoclonal antibodies which they provided and which Steve Mather radio-labelled. She continued at St Barts becoming a Reader in Nuclear Medicine of the University of London, except for 1 year when she was locum Consultant at the Middlesex Hospital in 1981, while Dr now Professor Peter Ell was in Berne. ICRF also supported technical staff notably Ms Sally Bentley and Mr Greg Morris, based with her at St Marks Hospital. Her research there with Professor John Northover using Tc-99m PR1A3 successfully detected recurrent colorectal cancer prior to surgery.

Her studies using Tc-99m HMFG1 or SM3 with Professor John Shepherd in Ovarian cancer and with Mr Rob Carpenter in Breast cancer were beneficial. Impalpable but involved axillary nodes were demonstrated prior to surgery. The analysis was aided by Cyril Nimmon's Probability Mapping computer programmes. All this work was presented at international meetings and published in peer-reviewed journals.

In-111 PSMA from Cytogen Corp. USA was first used by us in Europe to evaluate Prostate cancer recurrences with Mr Vinod Nargund. Applying Melvyn Carroll's advanced image analysis, the results were very encouraging and now Ga-68 PSMA is being introduced more widely.

11.4   EANM

It was created partly through Professor Erkki Vauramo's 'Sauna diplomacy' at the Finnish European Congress in 1984. The presidents of the two existing societies, the Society of Nuclear Medicine, Europe, SNME and the European Society of Nuclear Medicine, ESNM were incarcerated in the hot Sauna until they had reached a provisional agreement. As President of the SNME, I chaired a subsequent 'Linking Committee', a long meeting between the senior officers of the two societies. A draft constitution separating the powers of National Delegates and individual Members was initiated and I proposed the name. The first joint meeting of the two societies was held in 1985 at the Barbican Arts Centre, London, when I was Congress President and led the organising committee. We expected 1200 and over 3000 participants came. Ms Sue Hatchard, Secretary of the BNMS and her team organised the registration and paper work, Dr Ralph McCready sorted out the exhibition and the Trade Unions; Dr Reg Jewkes dealt with the finances, Dr Peter Ell took us to the theatre to see 42nd Street, Dr Keith Harding was front of house and Dr Andrew Hilson made the music happen for the opening ceremony with the Right Honourable Edward Heath, the speaker in the interval. He spoke of how Europe was like the Orchestra, made up of many nationalities and instruments, yet working together harmoniously – times have changed! We had dinner in the Great Hall of St Bartholomew's Hospital, Fig. 11.1.

'25 years of the EANM', contains a facsimile of the original contract. Clause 4 states that 'The European Association of Nuclear Medicine is founded in London at the European Nuclear Medicine Congress 1985 by the signatories of the contract' of whom I was one of the four, two from each Society. This makes our 1985 Congress in effect the first EANM meeting, even if it was not so titled.

11.5   Other Collaborative Work

Oncology with Professor Andrew Lister and Neuroendocrinology tumours, NETs, with Professor G. Michael Besser allowed us to develop or use new therapeutic agents. One of the most risky was the manufacture in house of I-131 MIBG for imaging and therapy. It required a 150 °C oil bath and large amounts of liquid I-131. It was undertaken by Laurie Hawkins and Dr Tipha Horne. We administered Y-90 Octreotide and Y-90 Lanreotide for NETs and Y-90 Bexxar anti-Lymphoma antibody for Non-Hodgkins disease. At St Marks we used P-32-PR1A3 for hepatic artery infusion for liver metastases with Angiotensin II administered to constrict the normal vessels; and intravenous P-32 labelled non-specific antibody at St Barts to target the bone marrow for the treatment of Polycythaemia.

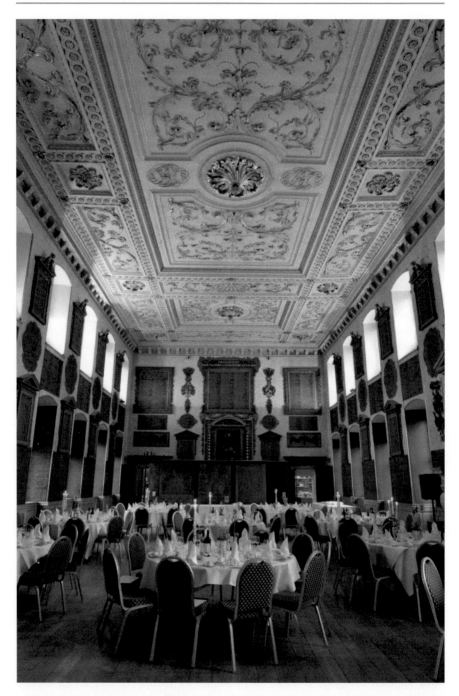

Fig. 11.1 The Great Hall at St Bartholomew's Hospital, set for dinner and overseen by Holbein's King Henry VIII at the head (Photograph courtesy of Joe D Miles, ImageCapture)

Cardiology was keenly developed with Dr Duncan Dymond. We had the first multi-crystal Baird Atomic camera in the UK. Most daring was using Gold Au-195m (Half-life 31 s) eluted from a Mercury column with dilute Cyanide, real alchemy! Alex Elliott was the brave volunteer for the first injection with Methylene Blue standing by. The first pass images showed beautiful, moment by moment, cardiac contraction and relaxation. The short half-life enabled repeat imaging every few minutes.

Myocardial Perfusion studies with SPECT followed and in 2 years we earned £1 million for the Trust for patients coming in from around the region. The administrators said we were charging too much to their customers and made us charge less than the cost of the procedure. Of course they then complained when we were over budget. There is no space to go into the troubles caused by administrators, I will just record that when I arrived there was one administrator to four nurses, when I left there were four administrators to one nurse. When I arrived there were over 800 beds, when I left there were under 400. As a result there were patients on trolleys in passages by Casualty waiting for beds. We Physicians called them 'Bottomley' wards after the Right Honourable Mrs Virginia Bottomley, who tried to close St Barts. She failed due to the courageous efforts of Professor Michael Besser and Dame Lesley Rees.

11.6   The Present and Future

I was made to retire due to age 65 in 2004. After a year's interregnum presumably to save the hospital money, Dr Norbert Avril was appointed in 2005 for his PET experience. A PET/CT, which I had requested, arrived in 2008 after a 5 year delay. Dr then Professor Avril ran it. He left in 2012. Dr Hikmat Jan, who had done the MSc with us in 1997 was appointed Clinical Lead. The research and postgraduate students returned with his enthusiasm. Dr Hikmat Jan and Ms Margaret Newell, Lead Physicist at the Royal London Hospital, designed the new department. It was opened at St Barts in 2014 in the basement of the totally new building behind the King George V frontage, a listed building.

The clinical staff became jointly responsible for the Nuclear Medicine at the Royal London Hospital after the long and excellent reign of Dr Neil Garvie, who retired in 2007. Recently they provide a service for Whipps Cross and Newham Hospitals and thus serve four sites. These are fully equipped with 7 gamma cameras in total with the one PET/CT at St Barts and are linked through a Hermes system.

The current Consultant staff are: Doctors Hikmat Jan, Lead Nuclear Medicine Physician, Lorenzo Biassoni, Ewa Nowosinska, Nuclear Medicine Physicians, Athar Haroon, Ayshea Hameeduddin, Yen Zhi Tang, Arman Parsai, Nuclear Medicine/Radiologists. A further Consultant Nuclear Medicine/Radiologist is due to be appointed in September 2015. They are supported by Chief Pharmacist Dr Neil Hartman from 2003 and his staff (now supplying six hospitals) and Lead Physicist Mrs Margaret Newell from 1976 with her staff and an excellent body of technologists. There are in training six Radiology registrars and three Foundation

Year 2 doctors. The annual work load has increased to over 4000 Myocardial Perfusion Studies and more than 2400 PET/CT. There is a growing SPECT/CT demand with the other general Nuclear Medicine procedures. New therapies include Lu-177 Dotatate for NETs, Radium-223 for bone metastases and Y-90 Theraspheres for liver tumours by intra hepatic artery infusion, while the traditional Iodine-131 based therapies continue.

Under its present active leadership, Nuclear Medicine in the St Barts and the London Trust is thriving and blossoming.

Keith Britton MSc MD FRCR FRCP
Emeritus Professor, University of London

Nuclear Medicine at the Hammersmith Hospital

12

Michael Peters

Nuclear medicine at the Hammersmith Hospital was established as a separate unit by Peter Lavender in the early seventies. It was called the Radioisotope Unit to distinguish it from the pre-existing Department of Medical Physics, headed by Harold Glass who was one of the early pioneers in medical radioisotope scanners [1]. As well as providing a clinical service, the unit, which only comprised two rooms, was active in clinical research complemented by the extensive academic activities of the MRC Cyclotron Unit. Two good examples of these activities that launched nuclear medicine at Hammersmith are firstly the development by Clark, Watson Fazio and Jones of Kr-81m for ventilation and perfusion studies [2], and secondly, cell labelling.

Kr-81m is a 13 s half-life radionuclide that is the metastable daughter of Rb-81, which has a half-life of 4.7 h. To obtain Kr-81m gas, oxygen is passed through the generator. There was an enthusiastic response to the generator across the UK, and, at one point, Kr-81m/Tc-99m ventilation/perfusion imaging was the second most frequently performed imaging procedure in the UK after bone scanning. Whilst Kr-81m remains the optimal ventilation agent for lung scanning, it is not so widely appreciated that Lavender and his colleagues also administered Kr-81 in solution to measure tissue perfusion. To obtain Kr-81m in solution, isotonic glucose is passed through the generator. For example, Harvey-Turner and Selwyn infused Kr-81m into the aortic root of dogs and continuously imaged regional changes in myocardial perfusion in response to transient coronary artery occlusion [3]. The distribution of pulmonary blood flow in humans was also imaged by continuous intravenous infusion [4]. Kr-81m was given both by inhalation and infusion to study ventilation-perfusion ratios and regional lung function in adults [4, 5] and children [6], When combined with the longer half-life Kr-85 (a lung gas volume marker), regional lung

M. Peters
Department of Nuclear Medicine, Clinical and Laboratory Investigation, Brighton and Sussex Medical School, Brighton BN1 9PX, UK

© The Author(s) 2016
R. McCready et al. (eds.), *A History of Radionuclide Studies in the UK:*
50th Anniversary of the British Nuclear Medicine Society,
DOI 10.1007/978-3-319-28624-2_12

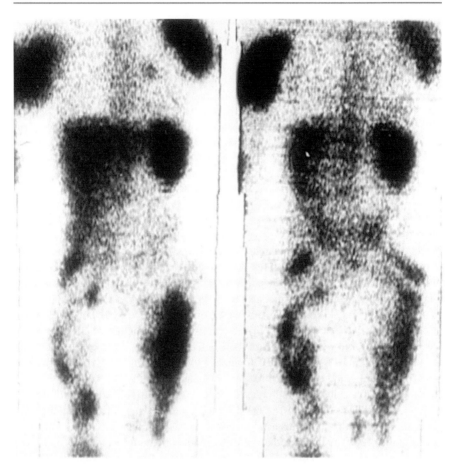

Fig. 12.1 A patient with multiple sites of sepsis imaged with In-111-labelled leucocytes (From Ref. [8])

function per unit volume could be assessed. Lavender used Kr-81m/Tc-99m SPECT in the early eighties to study pulmonary physiology [7] but did not feel that it offered any great advantage over planar imaging for diagnosing pulmonary thromboembolic disease.

The second example of innovative collaboration between Hammersmith nuclear medicine and MRC Cyclotron Unit was the development of cell labelling by Thakur and McAfee. John McAfee came to the Hammersmith for a 6 month sabbatical with the specific aim of working with Matthew Thakur to develop cell labelling for clinical imaging. Cr-51 had already been developed for cell labelling but is not suitable for gamma camera imaging, only surface counting. Testing several combinations of lipophilic chelating agents and radiometals, Thakur and McAfee came up with In-111 and hydroxyquinoline (oxine). The first full paper on leucocyte scanning for sepsis, based on 15 patients, was published in 1977 ([8]; Fig. 12.1).

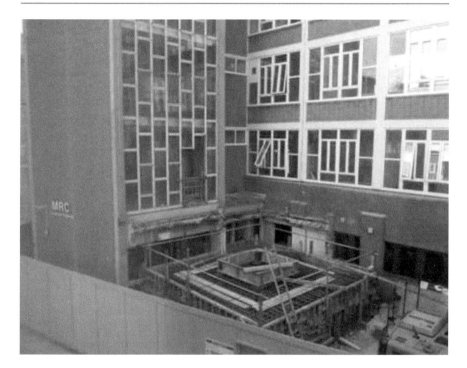

Fig. 12.2   The cyclotron being installed in the MRC building at the Hammersmith Hospital in 1956

There was great hope for performing labelled lymphocyte studies too, until it was soon found that lymphocytes are radio-sensitive and destroyed by labelling with amounts of In-111 required for imaging. I arrived at the Hammersmith in 1979 to undertake a 3-year Cancer Research Campaign-funded project on labelled lymphocytes but with this discovery quickly turned my attention to labelled leucocytes and platelets. In those days, Amersham International was not selling In-111-oxine, so it had to be prepared in-house (by a radio-chemist, Malcolm Kensett, in the MRC Cyclotron Unit). Once a patient had been identified, I would order the In-111-oxine, go to the MRC to collect it, take the patient's blood, go to the Haematology Isotope Unit to label it, then take it back to the Radioisotope Unit to inject it and image the patient. The Haematology isotope unit under the leadership of Mitchell Lewis, provided a tertiary service for ferrokinetics, using Fe-59 and Fe-52 (a positron emitter), and red cell survival and surface counting studies using Cr-51-labelled red cells. The unit also supported studies involving labelled cells, including In-111-labelled platelet kinetic studies by Klonikakis et al. [9], In-113m-labelled red cells and platelets, and studies on the clearance rates of labelled red cells modified by heating or antibody coating, undertaken by several workers from the Department of Medicine studying reticulo-endothelial (RE) function.

The Medical Research Council funded the building of a medical cyclotron on the Hammersmith site in 1954 (Fig. 12.2). This stimulated much research into cardiopulmonary physiology and neuro-pathophysiology in collaboration with the clinical staff of the Hospital. Pairs of scintillation detectors (front and back) were used first (with coincidence counting of positron emission), then planar gamma camera imaging, and finally positron emission tomography. The first studies were carried out in the late 1950s by West and his colleagues [10–12] using the short-lived positron emitting isotope, oxygen-15 (half life 2.1 min) as $C^{15}O_2$ and $C^{15}O$. Lung water distribution was studied with $H_2^{15}O$ [13, 14], pulmonary perfusion with infused $^{13}N_2$ in solution [15], pulmonary haemorrhage with inhaled ^{11}CO [16], and ventilation with neon-19 [17]. Rhodes and Hughes [18] summarized pulmonary studies using the positron camera. There was also much interest in studies of inflammatory conditions using F-18-fluorodeoxyglucose (^{18}FDG) [19, 20], and in imaging beta-agonist receptors in the heart and lung [21, 22].

Research activity elsewhere in the MRC Cyclotron Unit included the development of ^{18}FDG for imaging the brain (Terry Jones and Richard Frackowiak) and myocardium. Camici et al. were one of the first groups to image Rb-82 uptake in the myocardium of patients with coronary disease and show increased FDG uptake in ischaemic regions [23].

Many pioneers in nuclear medicine worked at Hammersmith. One of the earliest was Charles Galasko who in bone scintigraphy showed in 1968 that 12 of 50 patients with apparently 'early' breast cancer on clinical, radiological and biochemical grounds had positive scintigraphy and developed metastatic disease in the first 5 years following mastectomy [24]. Joseph Pflug was a pioneer in lymphatic function studies and was one of the first to use lymphoscintigraphy. Aga Epenetos, an oncologist, was one of the first to develop radiolabelled monocloncal antibodies for imaging cancer. Having worked with Keith Britton at St Bartholomew's and Walter Bodmer from the then ICRF, Epenetos continued his work at the Hammersmith. Also collaborating with ICRF, Lavender used a very effective monoclonal antibody to the platelet fibrinogen receptor for imaging thrombus ([25]; Fig. 12.3).

Dominic Haskard came to Hammersmith from Guy's Hospital around 1990 and developed very effective monocloncal antibodies to vascular adhesion molecules for imaging inflammation [26]. Sadly, however, none of these labelled antibodies made it into regular nuclear medicine practice.

Having developed In-111-oxine cell labelling, workers at the Hammersmith, again in collaboration with the MRC Cyclotron Unit (Danpure and Osman), then explored other chelating agents and discovered tropolone [27], which, now that GE do not offer In-111-oxine, is the standard agent for In-111 cell labelling. We then went on to develop Tc-99m-HMPAO for leucocyte labelling [28]. Saverymuttu demonstrated the extraordinary ability of In-111 and Tc-99m-labelled leucocyte scintigraphy to quantify and image inflammatory bowel disease (Fig. 12.4) and published numerous papers on its applications in gastroenterology.

Other, generally unfunded work, on patient volunteers established the normal whole body kinetics and physiological margination sites of granulocytes, and, in particular, dismantled the erroneous notion that the vast majority of intravascular granulocytes are pooled in the lungs [29]. It was clearly demonstrated how in systemic inflammatory diseases, such as pancreatitis, IBD and vasculitis, circulating granulocytes become primed, lose deformability and undergo prolonged transit through the pulmonary vasculature. This is in contrast to hold-up in the lungs of

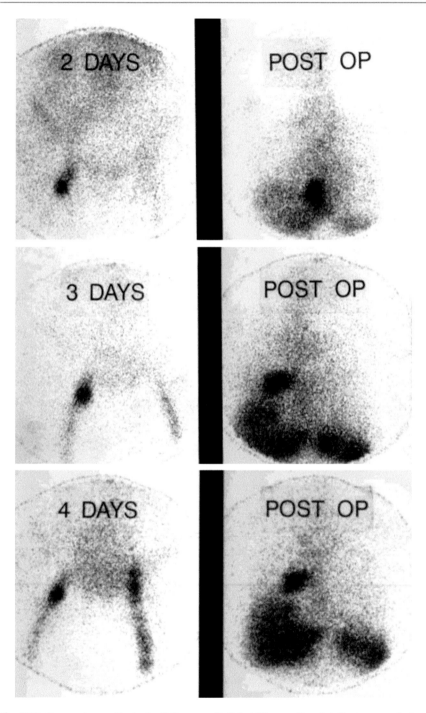

Fig. 12.3 Images in a patient who 2 (*top panel*), 3 (*middle panel*) and 4 (*bottom panel*) days before receiving a total hip replacement. The In-111-labelled antibody P256 was administered shortly after surgery. Note the development of thrombus in the femoral veins and the movement of an embolus from the right ventricle to right pulmonary artery (From Ref. [25])

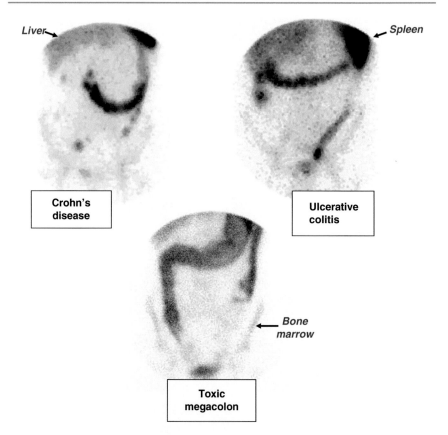

Fig. 12.4 Inflammatory bowel disease imaged 1 h after injection of Tc-99m-HMPAO-labelled leucocytes

granulocytes artificially activated by the labelling procedure and associated with very low intravascular recovery. This work led to quality control guidelines for leucocyte labelling.

Another major nuclear medicine landmark in the history of the Hammersmith radioisotope unit was the development by Mark Pepys and Philip Hawkins of I-123-labelled serum amyloid protein (SAP) for imaging amyloidosis [30]. This work was dramatically successful and led to the establishment of a separate unit in the hospital with its own gamma camera and technical staff, such was the weight of referrals from all over the country. So, at one time, there were five separate nuclear medicine units on the Hammersmith site! I remember Pepys and Hawkins opening champagne in the Radioisotope Unit when they had just witnessed heavy hepatic uptake of labelled SAP in a patient with amyloidosis (Fig. 12.5). I wondered if the celebrations might be premature, having learned that in general when a tracer is not functioning properly it is liable to end up in the liver, but this was clearly not the case!

The spirit of research collaboration at the Hammersmith Hospital fuelled many interesting research projects using radionuclides. For example, the early advances in

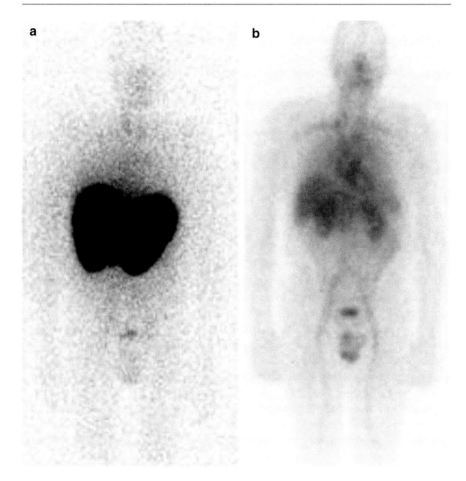

Fig. 12.5 Hepato-splenic amyloidosis (**a**) compared with normal distribution of I-123-labelled SAP (**b**) (From Refs. [29])

interventional radiology allowed us to inject In-111-labelled platelets directly into the splenic artery of patients having arterial catheterization and show conclusively that platelets pool in the spleen and are released after a mean residence time of about 10 min. Plasma exchange for the treatment of immune complex disease was shown to be associated with improved RE function as measured by the splenic extraction efficiency of radiolabelled antibody-coated red cells, using simultaneously injected In-111-labelled platelets to measure splenic blood flow [31]. Before then, it had been thought that RE function could be quantified by the clearance rate of heat-damaged red cells until we showed that the clearance rate reflected splenic pooling and was therefore, like platelet equilibration between blood and spleen, a measure of splenic blood flow. Early studies on pulmonary epithelial permeability using inhaled Tc-99m-DTPA [32] and pulmonary endothelial permeability using intravenous In-111-transferrin [33] were performed by Royston and his co-workers. Davies and Walport demonstrated for the first time the whole body kinetics of I-123-labelled immune complexes [34].

In the mid-nineties, rotaPET was acquired by what had now been re-named the 'Nuclear Medicine Department'. This was a partial ring detector consisting of two separate segments and was used predominantly for FDG imaging of cancer but also clinical F-18-DOPA brain imaging. The department was involved in early clinical work with In-111-pentetriotide and showed how amino acid infusion blocked renal tubular uptake of the agent [35]. In research, Harrington and Stewart demonstrated the targeting of tumours by In-111-labelled stealth liposomes containing chemotherapeutic agents [36]. In collaboration with 'Tiny' Maini from the Institute of Rheumatology, the therapeutic effect of TNFα blockade was shown to reduce dramatically leucocyte uptake in rheumatoid joints [37]. Muhammad Mubashar was one of the first workers to image P-glycoprotein expression in breast cancer [38]. As one of the first centres in the UK to develop interventional radiology, the Hammersmith Hospital was a referral centre for conditions such as pulmonary arterio-venous shunts and much work with the Department of Respiratory Medicine [39] was performed to quantify these shunts before and after therapeutic embolization. Finally, elegant work performed in collaboration with George Hall, an anaesthetist with an interest in exercise physiology, demonstrated in trained athletes undergoing maximal brief exercise how platelets and all leucocyte subtypes pool in the spleen with similar residence times [40]. Contrasting the behaviour of red cells versus leucocytes and platelets in response to exercise, he showed that the spleen is essentially an erectile organ – permanently erect!

In the time I was at Hammersmith Hospital (1979–1999), the Hammersmith campus was probably the leading medical research hospital in the UK, and enjoyed a reputation based on a fantastic multidisciplinary approach and spirit of collaboration, co-operation and clinical support. Clinical research in nuclear medicine that goes beyond the evaluation of the latest novel radiopharmaceutical or imaging hardware critically depends on support from the clinicians, and this support was second-to-none at the Hammersmith.

Acknowledgements The author would like to thank Prof Mike Hughes and Prof Peter Lavender for advice regarding the work described in this article.

References

1. Glass HI, Hudson FR, French MT. A 70 mm diameter germanium detector medical radioisotope scanner. Medical Radioisotope Scintigraphy. Vienna: IAEA; 1973.
2. Fazio F, Jones T. Assessment of regional ventilation by continuous inhalation of radioactive krypton-81m. Br Med J. 1975;3(5985):673–6.
3. Turner JH, Selwyn AP, Jones T, et al. Continuous imaging of regional myocardial blood flow in dogs using krypton-81m. Cardiovasc Res. 1976;10:398–404.
4. Harf A, Pratt T, Hughes JMB. Regional distribution of VA/Q in man at rest and on exercise measured with krypton-81m. J Appl Physiol. 1978;44:115–23.
5. Amis TC, Jones HA, Hughes JMB. Effect of posture on interregional distribution of pulmonary perfusion and VA/Q ratios in man. Respir Physiol. 1984;56:169–82.
6. Ciofetta G, Silverman M, Hughes JMB. Quantitative approach to the study of regional lung function in children using Krypton-81m. Br J Radiol. 1980;53:950–9.
7. Lavender JP, Al-Nahhas AM, Myers MJ. Ventilation perfusion ratios of the normal supine lung using emission tomography. Br J Radiol. 1984;57:141–6.
8. Thakur ML, Lavender JP, Arnot RN, et al. Indium-111-labeled autologous leukocytes in man. J Nucl Med. 1977;18:1014–21.
9. Klonizakis I, Peters AM, Fitzpatrick ML, et al. Radionuclide distribution following injection of indium-111 labelled platelets. Br J Haematol. 1980;46:595–602.
10. West JB, Dollery CT. Distribution of blood flow and ventilation-perfusion ratio in the lung, measured with radioactive CO_2. J Appl Physiol. 1960;15:405–10.
11. West JB, Dollery CT. Absorption of inhaled radioactive water vapour. Nature. 1961;189:588.
12. West JB, Dollery CT, Hugh-Jones P. The use of radioactive carbon dioxide to measure regional blood flow in the lungs of patients with pulmonary disease. J Clin Invest. 1961;40:1–12.
13. Jones T, Jones HA, Rhodes CG, et al. Distribution of extravascular fluid volumes in isolated perfused lungs measured with $H_2{}^{15}O$. J Clin Invest. 1976;57:706–13.
14. Swinburne AJ, MacArthur CGC, Rhodes CG, et al. Measurement of lung water in dog lobes using inhaled $C^{15}O_2$ and injected $H_2{}^{15}O$. J Appl Physiol Respir Environ Exercise Physiol. 1982;52:1535–44.
15. Ewan PW, Jones HA, Nosil J, et al. Uneven perfusion and ventilation within lung regions studied with nitrogen-13. Respir Physiol. 1976;34:45–60.
16. Ewan PW, Jones HA, Rhodes CG, et al. Detection of intrapulmonary haemorrhage with carbon monoxide uptake: application in Goodpasture's Syndrome. N Engl J Med. 1976;295:1391–6.
17. Valind SO, Rhodes CG, Brudin LH, et al. Measurements of regional ventilation pulmonary gas volume: theory and error analysis with special reference to positron emission tomography. J Nucl Med. 1991;32:1937–44.
18. Rhodes CG, Hughes JMB. Pulmonary studies using positron emission tomography. Eur Respir J. 1995;8:1001–17.
19. Jones HA, Clark RJ, Rhodes CG, et al. In vivo measurement of neutrophil activity in experimental lung inflammation. Am J Respir Crit Care Med. 1994;149:1635–9.
20. Jones HA. Inflammation imaging. Proc Am Thorac Soc. 2005;513–4:545–8.
21. Ueki J, Rhodes CG, Hughes JMB, et al. In vivo quantification of pulmonary beta-adrenoceptor density in man u sing S[^{11}C]CGP12177 and positron emission tomography. J Appl Physiol. 1993;75:559–65.
22. Hayes MJ, Qing F, Rhodes CG, et al. *In vivo* quantification of human pulmonary β-adrenoceptors with PET: effect of β-agonist therapy. Am J Resp Crit Care Med. 1996;154:1277–83.
23. Camici P, Araujo LI, Spinks T, et al. Increased uptake of ^{18}F-fluorodeoxyglucose in postischemic myocardium of patients with exercise-induced angina. Circulation. 1986;74:81–8.
24. Galasko CS, Westerman B, Sellwood RA, et al. Use of the gamma camera for early detection of osseous metastases from mammary cancer. Br J Surg. 1968;55:613–5.

25. Peters AM, Lavender JP, Needham SG, et al. Imaging thrombus with a radiolabelled monoclonal antibody to platelets. Br Med J. 1986;293:1525–7.
26. Jamar F, Chapman PT, Harrison AA, et al. Inflammatory arthritis: imaging of endothelial cell activation with an In-111 labeled F(ab')$_2$ fragment of anti-E-selectin monoclonal antibody. Radiology. 1995;194:843–50.
27. Peters AM, Saverymuttu SH, Reavy HJ, et al. Imaging inflammation with 111-indium tropolonate labeled leukocytes. J Nucl Med. 1983;24:39–44.
28. Peters AM, Danpure HJ, Osman S, et al. Preliminary clinical experience with Tc-99m-HMPAO for labelling leucocytes and imaging inflammation. Lancet. 1986;2:946–9.
29. Peters AM. Just how big is the pulmonary granulocyte pool? Clin Sci. 1998;94:7–19.
30. Hawkins PN, Myers MJ, Lavender JP, et al. Diagnostic radionuclide imaging of amyloid: biological targeting by circulating human serum amyloid P component. Lancet. 1988;1(8600):1413–8.
31. Walport MJ, Peters AM, Elkon KB, et al. The splenic extraction ratio of antibody coated erythrocytes and its response to plasma exchange and pulse methy-lprednisolone. Clin Exp Immunol. 1985;65:465–73.
32. Nolop KB, Maxwell DL, Fleming JS, et al. A comparison of ^{99m}Tc-DTPA and ^{113m}In-DTPA aerosol clearances in humans. Effects of smoking, hyperinflation and in vitro oxidation. Am Rev Respir Dis. 1987;136:1112–6.
33. Braude S, Nolop KB, Hughes JMB, et al. Comparison of lung vascular and epithelial permeability indices in the Adult Respiratory Distress Syndrome. Am Rev Respir Dis. 1986;133:1002–5.
34. Davies KA, Peters AM, Beynon HLC, et al. Immune complex processing in patients with sysytemic lupus erythematosus – in vivo imaging and clearance studies. J Clin Invest. 1992;90:2075–83.
35. Hammond PJ, Wade AF, Gwilliam ME, et al. Amino acid infusion blocks renal tubular uptake of an indium-labelled somatostatin analogue. Br J Cancer. 1993;67:1437–9.
36. Harrington KJ, Mohammadtaghi S, Uster PS, et al. Effective targeting of solid tumours in patients with locally advanced cancers by radiolabelled pegylated liposomes. Clin Cancer Res. 2001;7:243–54.
37. Taylor PC, Paleolog E, Chapman PT, et al. TNFα blockade in patients with rheumatoid arthritis reduces chemokines and leukocyte traffic to joints. Arthr Rheum. 2000;43:38–47.
38. Mubashar M, Harrington KJ, Chaudhary KS, et al. Tc-99m-sestamibi imaging in the assessment of toremifene as a modulator of multidrug resistance in patients with breast cancer. J Nucl Med. 2002;43:519–25.
39. Whyte MKB, Peters AM, Hughes JMB, et al. Quantification of right-to-left shunt at rest and during exercise in patients with pulmonary arteriovenous malformations. Thorax. 1992;47:790–6.
40. Allsop P, Peters AM, Arnot RN, et al. Intrasplenic blood cell kinetics in man before and after brief maximal exercise. Clin Sci. 1992;83:47–54.

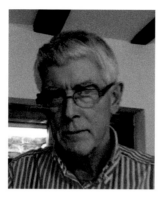

Michael Peters I did my pre-clinical training at St Mary's Hospital Medical School where I received a BSc in physiology in 1967. I then transferred to Liverpool University and received MB ChB in 1970. In 1972, I was appointed as lecturer in physiology in the medical school at Liverpool. This is where I discovered my interest in the use of radionuclides to study human physiology and did an MD in the use of Xenon-133 to measure hepatic perfusion. Uncertain of what I then wanted to do, I went to Australia and became a GP for 4 years, doing many different jobs and discovering the attractions of the country. I returned to England in 1978 a few weeks before my mother succumbed to breast cancer, and after a year in general practice in Liverpool 8 secured a clinical research fellowship at the Royal Postgraduate Medical School to work on In-111-labelled lymphocytes. There I met my mentor, Peter Lavender, and the great Robert Steiner. There followed 3 years of intense research on In-111 cell labelling and then the funding ran out so I joined Glaxo Group Research as a Research Physician. My big break came in 1984 when Isky Gordon and Peter Lavender created a senior lectureship in radiology split between RPMS and the Institute of Child Health. These two great functional radiologists convinced me of the importance of integrated imaging, a view later cemented by the introduction of PACS at the Hammersmith Hospital in the mid-nineties. In 1988, I became full time at RPMS and then, with Peter's retirement in 1991, ran nuclear medicine at Hammersmith single-handedly until 1999 when I was appointed Foundation Professor of Nuclear Medicine in Cambridge. At this time, Cambridge Medical School was growing rapidly under the leadership of Keith Peters, a man I greatly admired when he was Professor of Medicine at RPMS. I spent 6 productive years in Cambridge, working with Edwin Chilvers (respiratory medicine) and Arnie Purushotham (breast cancer), before moving to the new medical school in Brighton. The first appointments made in Brighton were Jon Cohen as Dean and Kevin Davies as Professor of Medicine, both ex Hammersmith colleagues, so whilst Cambridge was jokingly called Hammersmith North, Brighton became known as Hammersmith South. I should have retired 5 years ago but I am still working full-time and enjoying the research as much as ever. The three high points of my career were election to the fellowship of the Academy of Medical Sciences in 2002, award of a DSc from the University of Liverpool in 2009 and invitation to give the Annual Lecture at the spring meeting of the BNMS in Brighton in 2011.

Nuclear Medicine in Nottingham: Antibodies, Gamma Probes and Drug Delivery

13

Alan C. Perkins

When I started work in Nottingham in 1980 University Hospital had only recently been built. The University of Nottingham Medical School and Hospital was officially opened by the Queen on 28 July 1977 and named 'Queen's Medical Centre'. At the time it was completed it was to be one of the biggest hospitals in Europe with over 1300 beds and 27 miles of corridor. The nuclear medicine department was equipped with a Siemens single head camera and was the first out patient department in the hospital to receive patients. This was one of three hospitals in Nottingham where nuclear medicine was undertaken, the other two being Nottingham City Hospital and the Nottingham General Hospital near Standard Hill, (named after the point where King Charles raised his Royal Standard in 1642, thus starting the English Civil War). In the early 1980s the General Hospital was still carrying out nuclear medicine scans on a rather old rectilinear scanner. When this facility was closed nuclear medicine was further developed at both Queen's Medical Centre and the Nottingham City Hospital. With the Medical School still being in its infancy there were many young clinical and scientific staff eager to make an impact and many diverse areas of research developed that involved nuclear medicine techniques.

The Cancer Research Laboratories at Nottingham University were a collection of old single story huts on the university site now occupied by the Biomedical Sciences Building, on the opposite side of the ring road to the Medical School. In the early 1980s Professor Robert Baldwin lead a team of 50 scientists who were developing the then new monoclonal antibody technology. Along with the University of Birmingham, and the Charring Cross Hospital, London, Nottingham pioneered the

A.C. Perkins
Department of Radiological Sciences, University of Nottingham, Nottingham, UK

Radiological Sciences, Nottingham University Hospitals NHS Trust, Nottingham, UK

© The Author(s) 2016
R. McCready et al. (eds.), *A History of Radionuclide Studies in the UK: 50th Anniversary of the British Nuclear Medicine Society*,
DOI 10.1007/978-3-319-28624-2_13

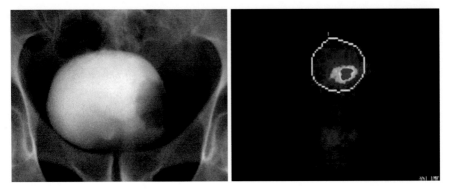

Fig. 13.1 An intravenous urogram and ^{67}Cu-C595 image in a patient with a superficial cancer of the bladder

in vivo use of monoclonal antibody imaging. One of the first antibodies to be used was 791t/36 produced from a patient with osteogenic sarcoma. The first clinical use of this antibody was carried out in patients with colorectal cancer [1]. The imaging was technically demanding since the first antibodies were radiolabelled with I-131 and the long survival of the antibody in the circulation necessitated the use of background subtraction employing Tc-99m-labelled human serum albumin [2]. The work with monoclonal antibodies progressed with Nottingham undertaking some of the first in vivo studies using In-111 and Tc-99m-labelled antibodies [3, 4] and published one of the first studies of SPECT antibody imaging [5]. Work with antibody fragments (Fab and F(ab')2) progressed and over the next 10 years the affects of antibody responses were observed leading to a decline in routine use. Therapeutic trials of Cu-67-C595 anti-MUC1 antibody in bladder cancer continued and this approach still offers unexplored potential Fig. 13.1 [6]. The European directives on the GMP conditions required for the production of biologicals including antibodies, meant that the Nottingham production facilities were no longer suitable for the manufacture of clinical grade materials and so the "home grown" antibody studies came to an end.

Other work in Nottingham led the way for the early use of intraoperative probes for the detection of lesions removed during surgery. Work started by John Hardy with one of the orthopaedic surgeons, Chris Colton in Nottingham led to the use of the gamma probe for the localization of osteoid osteoma Fig. 13.2 [7].

This pre-dated the use of gamma probes for sentinel node detection and led to the development of the RMD gamma probe in the United States. Over a period of 10 years I personally travelled from Southampton to Aberdeen assisting surgeons localize a variety of lesions [7, 8]. Similar techniques were developed for the use of probes in the intensive care unit [9].

Over the past 30 years Nottingham has been associated with other areas of nuclear medicine research. Working with Malcolm Frier a range of novel radiopharmaceutical products were developed and investigated including recombinant human

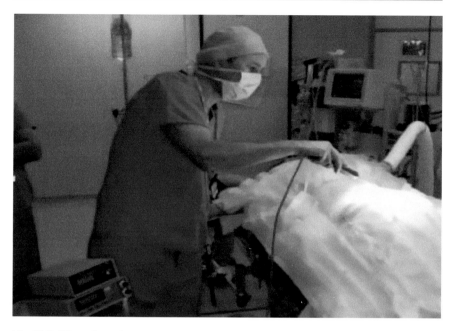

Fig. 13.2 The author using an early gamma probe in the operating theatre in the 1980s

serum albumin [10] a spin off from the Bass brewing industry and recombinant branched-chain polypeptide synthetics [11] and aptamers [12]. Perhaps more unique to Nottingham was the use of nuclear medicine techniques in the study of conventional drug delivery and formulation. Extensive studies were undertaken to image the release, delivery and biodistribution of formulations including enteric coated oral dose forms, enemas, eye drops, nasal sprays and aerosols [13–15]. Much of this work has involved the study of tablet swallowing [16], gastrointestinal transit, the understanding of gastrointestinal physiology and the development of nuclear medicine imaging techniques for the study of the gastrointestinal tract Fig. 13.3 [17].

These areas of work have continued with the application of magnetic resonance imaging in the study of gastrointestinal transit [18, 19].

More recently through a collaboration with John Lees at the Space Research Centre at Leicester University, Nottingham has been pioneering the first clinical use of a hand-held hybrid optical gamma camera for small parts imaging and for use in intraoperative imaging Fig. 13.4 [20]. Studies are continuing in collaboration with surgeons in Nottingham and Derby.

Acknowledgements I would like to express my appreciation to some of the many colleagues who I have worked with in Nottingham and who have helped in my career over the past 35 years. These include John Hardy, Jack Hardcastle, Clive Wilson, Bob Davies, Malcolm Pimm, Mike Price, Malcolm Symonds, Malcolm Frier, Colin Barber, Martin Wastie and John Lees.

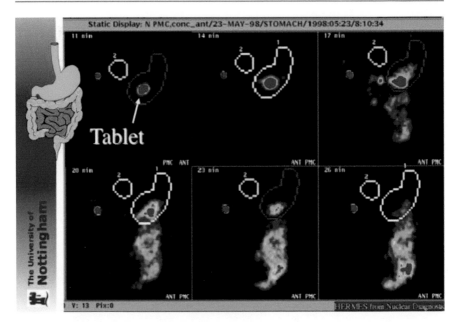

Fig. 13.3 Shows the process of a tablet in the stomach disintegrating and emptying into the small bowel

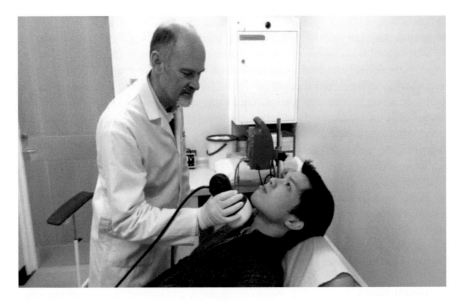

Fig. 13.4 A hand held intraoperative hybrid optical gamma camera

References

1. Farrands PA, Perkins AC, Pimm MV, Hardy JG, Baldwin RW, Hardcastle JD. Radioimmunodetection of human colorectal cancers using an anti-tumour monoclonal antibody. Lancet. 1982;II:397–400.
2. Perkins AC, Whalley DR, Hardy JG. Physical approach for the reduction of dual radionuclide image subtraction artefacts in immunoscintigraphy. Nucl Med Commun. 1984;5:501–12.
3. Perkins AC, Pimm MV, Birch MK. The preparation and characterisation of In-111-labelled 791T/36 monoclonal antibody for tumour immunoscintigraphy. Eur J Nucl Med. 1985;10:296–301.
4. Pimm MV, Perkins AC, Baldwin RW. Labelling of monoclonal antibody with metallic radionuclides: preparation of antibody-DTPA conjugates from DTPA anhydride in organic solvent. ICRS Med Sci. 1986;14:104–5.
5. Perkins AC, Whalley DR, Ballantyne KC, Pimm MV. Gamma camera emission tomography using radiolabelled antibodies. Eur J Nucl Med. 1988;14:45–9.
6. Hughes ODM, Bishop MC, Perkins AC, Wastie ML, Denton G, Price MR, Frier M, Denley H, Rutherford R, Scubiger PA. Targeting superficial bladder cancer by the intravesical administration of Cu-67-labelled anti-MUC1 mucin monoclonal antibody. J Clin Oncol. 2000;18:363–70.
7. Perkins AC, Hardy JG. Intra-operative nuclear medicine in surgical practice. Nucl Med Commun. 1996;17:1006–15.
8. Aslam A, Perkins AC, Spicer RD. Peroperative I-123-MIBG scan using a sterile probe for staging and resection of neuroblastoma in children. J Pediatr Surg. 1996;5:719–20.
9. Perkins AC, Yeoman P, Hindle AJ, Vincent RM, Frier M, Winter RJ, Wastie ML. Bedside nuclear medicine investigations in the intensive care unit. Nucl Med Commun. 1997;18:262–8.
10. Perkins AC, Frier M. Experimental biodistribution studies of Tc-99m-recombinant human serum albumin (rHSA); a new generation of radiopharmaceutical. Eur J Nucl Med. 1994;21:1231–3.
11. Perkins AC, Frier M, Pimm MV, Hudecz F. Tc-99m-branched-chain polypeptide (BCP): a potential synthetic radiopharmaceutical. J Labelled Compounds Radiopharm. 1998;XLI:631–8.
12. Perkins AC, Missailidis S. Radiolabelled aptamers for tumour imaging and therapy. Q J Nucl Med Mol Imaging. 2007;51:1–5.
13. Perkins AC, Pimm MV, Wilson CG. Gamma scintigraphy in the delivery, biodistribution and targeting of therapeutic agents. J Nucl Biol Med. 1994;38(Suppl 1 to No 4):113–8.
14. Perkins AC, Frier M. Nuclear medicine in pharmaceutical research. London: Taylor and Francis; 1999.
15. Perkins AC, Frier M. Radionuclide imaging in drug development. Curr Pharm Design. 2004;10:2907–21.
16. Frier M, Perkins AC. Radiopharmaceuticals and the gastrointestinal tract. Eur J Nucl Med. 1994;21:1234–42.
17. Perkins AC, Blackshaw PE, Hay PD, Lawes SC, Atherton CT, Dansereau RJ, Wagner LK, Schnell DJ, Spiller RC. Esophageal transit and in vivo disintegration of generic alendronate tablets and branded Risedronate tablets: a single-center, single-blind, six-period crossover study in 20 healthy female subjects. Clin Ther. 2008;30:834–44.

18. Yeong CH, Abdullah BJJ, K-H NG, Chung L-Y, Goh K-L, Perkins AC. Fusion of gamma scintigraphic and MR images improves the anatomical delineation of radiotracer for the assessment of gastrointestinal transit. Nucl Med Commun. 2013;34:645–51.
19. Chaddock G, Lam C, Hoad CL, Costigan C, Cox EF, Placidi E, Thexton I, Wright J, Blackshaw PE, Perkins AC, Marciani L, Gowland PA, Spiller RC. Novel MRI tests of orocecal transit time and whole gut transit time: studies in normal subjects. Neurogastroenterol Motil. 2014;26(2):205–14.
20. Lees JE, Bassford DJ, Blake OE, Blackshaw PE, Perkins AC. A hybrid camera for simultaneous imaging of gamma and optical photons. J IINST. 2012. doi:10.1088/1748-0221/7/06/P06009.

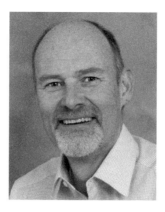

Alan Perkins After completing an MSc in Medical Physics at the University of Leeds in 1979 I started work in Medical Physics at Queen's Medical Centre, Nottingham, where I undertook a PhD in Monoclonal Antibody Imaging in the department of Surgery in the Medical School at the University of Nottingham from 1983 to 1986. After a period heading up Nuclear Medicine and Radiation Protection in the hospital department I took up a university post as Reader in Medical Physics and was appointed to Clinical Professor in 1999. I was awarded Fellow of the Institute of Physics and Engineering in Medicine in 1990, Fellow of the Royal College of Radiologists, in 2008 and an honorary Fellow of the Royal College of Physicians of London in 2011. During my time as President of the British Nuclear Medicine Society I helped establish the society offices to their current location at the Nottingham University Innovation Park.

The Introduction and Development of Clinical PET in the United Kingdom

14

Michael Maisey

Twenty-five years ago (half the life of the BNMS) in 1990 clinical PET imaging began to be accepted as an important clinical diagnostic tool (Fig. 14.1).

There were then approximately 60 pet centres in the United States 20 in Japan and even six in Belgium however there was not a single clinical PET service in the United Kingdom in spite of the fact that the Medical Cyclotron and PET unit at the Hammersmith Hospital was at the cutting edge of research in this area.

In 1990, during a post prandial stroll back to our hotel during EANM conference, Desmond Croft (Gastroenterologist and head of Nuclear Medicine at St Thomas' hospital) and I discussed the possibility of establishing the first clinical PET Centre in the UK. Guys and St Thomas' Medical schools had been united in 1984 to form the joint United Medical and Dental Schools (UMDS) but the two hospitals remained separate entities (although later merging to form one hospital trust) We felt at the time that a single PET centre supported by both hospitals and based in the medical school would make it more likely that we could raise the necessary support and critically the funding.

Looking back to that time Twenty-five years ago it is interesting to note that the proposal was based mainly on neuropsychiatric indications (predominantly to identify pre-surgical sites of focal epilepsy and early diagnosis of Alzheimer's disease) and Cardiological applications (viability of ischaemic compromised myocardium) there was some early evidence from the United States and elsewhere that applications in cancer might assume a greater importance which at that time was restricted mainly to brain tumour recurrence and some early work in staging and recurrent Lung cancer.

M. Maisey
Kings College, London, UK

© The Author(s) 2016
R. McCready et al. (eds.), *A History of Radionuclide Studies in the UK:
50th Anniversary of the British Nuclear Medicine Society*,
DOI 10.1007/978-3-319-28624-2_14

Fig. 14.1 Clinical PET
its time has come recorded
on the cover of the
*Journal of Nuclear
Medicine* in 1991

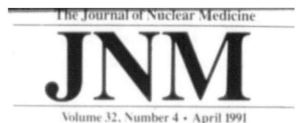

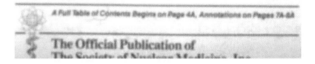

The concept we discussed that evening was to develop a clinical PET centre which was both a clinical service and a clinical research centre which would encompass a small medical cyclotron with a radiochemistry laboratory, with clinical PET scan imaging facilities at Guys hospital and St Thomas' Hospital with the whole centre functioning as a single entity. This plan seemed to make the likelihood of success higher as initial estimates suggested that around £5 million would need to be raised.

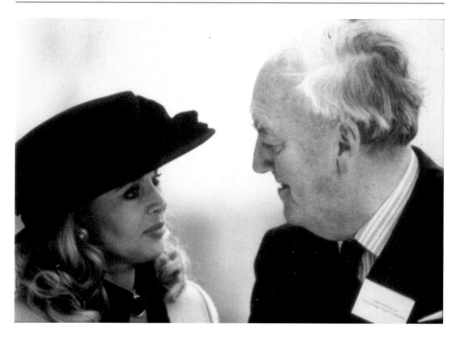

Fig. 14.2 Ex deputy prime minister under Margaret Thatcher-Lord William Whitelaw with Brit Ekland

The proposals were presented to UMDS and the boards of both Hospital Trusts and after considerable discussion the plan was supported by both the hospitals and Medical School with the new centre in the newly created division of Radiological Sciences. At that time Trusts were very separate from the academic school and were more risk adverse. The absolute 'proviso' was that we must raise the capital funding and the centre should be financially self supporting with all staff and running costs to be covered by charging for scan referrals, selling radiotracers from the radiochemistry unit as well as grants supporting clinical research projects.

After an initial period of planning and costing, with significant support from the Hammersmith PET group, even though there were some who did not believe that it was appropriate to use PET for clinical purposes! Early funding was raised from several sponsors before a formal fundraising program was established. We were fortunate in persuading the ex deputy prime minister under Margaret Thatcher-Lord William "every Prime Minister should have a Willie" Whitelaw to chair the appeal aptly named 'The Living Image appeal' Fig. 14.2.

The first formal meeting of which took place in December 1991 in the House of Lords! Lord Whitelaw proved to be an excellent chairman and within 6 months approximately 2.3 million had been raised and work to establish the centre was underway. The cyclotron itself was to be installed in the basement of St Thomas's Hospital with an imaging centre on the ground floor above and the second unit was incorporated in the physics Department below the nuclear medicine department at

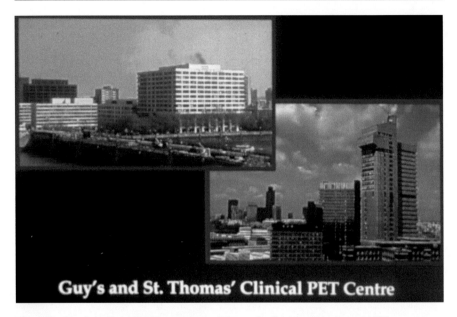

Fig. 14.3 The first clinical PET centre in the UK was finally opened in August 1992

Guys Hospital. Figure 14.3 shows St Thomas Hospital overlooking the river Thames on the left and Guy's Hospital tower on the right (Fig. 14.4).

During 1994 the 'Living image appeal' was discontinued as the total sum of £5 million had been reached and the centre was a going concern with significant external funded referrals and further income raised by selling cyclotron produced radiopharmaceuticals to increasing numbers of developing clinical PET facilities around the country. Added to this was the clinical research grants which had been gained.

It is interesting to note that by the end of the first year approximately 28 % of the clinical scans were referrals for cancer; diagnosis and treatment monitoring and by 1994 the figure had risen to 48 % currently the figure runs at over 90 %. Around half of the scans were for clinical purposes and approximately half for funded clinical research projects and all staff and running costs were being covered by the income from these sources. On the basis of our original projections (Neuropsychiatric and Cardiac) it has to be doubted whether the project would have been financially viable, but that is now history.

It is difficult to overestimate the importance of an effective team, with no formal training, to run a unit of this type, both then and now. Everybody: administrative, technical, radiographers scientists (Physics, Chemists and Computer scientists) as well as doctors, were essential and remain essential to the effective working of a unit of this type. Twenty-five years ago it was a very steep learning curve for everyone involved, particularly for the medical staff for whom formal training in clinical PET was not generally available. Also there was little available in the literature this meant learning and reporting the appearances of abnormal PET scans equally important was learning the range of normal variations of the physiological

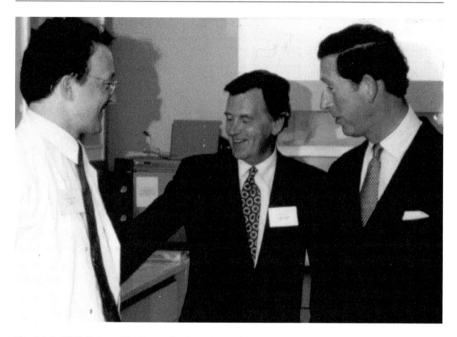

Fig. 14.4 HRH Prince Charles at the formal opening of the Clinical PET centre. Prof Michael Maisey and Dr Tony Gee, Radio chemist demonstrates the equipment to Prince Charles on the *right*

distribution of tracer. A significant innovation in organisation was the blind double reading whereby each scan was read independently, disagreements discussed and agreed upon or referred to a third reader. I believe using this method we moved up the learning curve more rapidly and avoided many potentially serious errors: an arrangement which continues today.

Although we had expected to be mainly involved in neuropsychiatric and Cardiological applications it became clear that cancer would form a huge amount of the workload of clinical PET and this has continued. It was always expected that a range of biological traces would be involved however the fundamental tracer Fluoro-deoxy Glucose (FDG) proved to be by far the most important and remains so today.

Gradually with the clinical success from referrals many other centres invested in PET imaging devices, as long as it was possible to obtain the appropriate tracers without the necessity of establishing at cyclotron and a radiochemistry unit the costs could be kept down there are now medical cyclotrons and diagnostic PET units in the UK many of which are commercial subcontracted to NHS of which about half are mobile systems including two suppliers of PET tracers (FDG, F-Choline and 18F Fluoride).

Anatomic localisation of the sites of tracer uptake in around 10 % of the cases remained a clinical problem for reporting scans. Early research work, in conjunction with our Radiological sciences computer imaging group, combining PET images with more conventional CT and MRI images Fig. 14.5 based on computer-generated image fusion was productive.

This image fusion, of course, was later taken on by the commercial manufacturers incorporating CT and later MR into the imaging device itself (PET/CT) which

Fig. 14.5 PET and CT
fused image of the skull

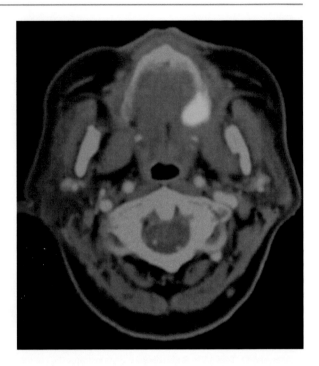

permitted accurate localisation as well as quicker attenuation correction, 8 patients/
day was then maximum throughput, now about twice that rate is possible. The vast
majority of PET devices are now PET CT devices and a few, including a new one at
the Guys St Thomas's PET centre, incorporate MRI (PET/MR). This has also meant
that non radiology trained Nuclear Medicine staff have had to undertake more formal training in cross sectional anatomical imaging.

The future remains exciting with further development of specific radio traces, in
addition to FDG: F-Choline is routine for prostate cancer, 68Gallium for neuroendocrine tumours and 68Gallium PSMA has just become commercially available. An
area that we thought at the time would be important; combined PET and MR spectroscopy has not as yet delivered any significant advances.

In 2015 25 years after the start of the first UK PET centre the whole unit has
been refurbished with 2 new PET/CT scanners and a high field 3 T PET/MR
scanner for clinical and basic research including spectroscopy. There is a PET /
CT planned for the new cancer centre in 2016. In addition cyclotron and chemistry laboratories are being refurbished and is now probably the best equipped
and most productive unit in the UK and I'm proud to have been associated with
the onset and introduction of clinical PET into the United Kingdom. Research
continues to be of great importance and a short selection of some key research
publications below.

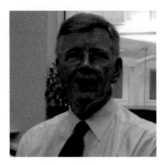

Michael Maisey After completing an MD based on an 131 biological assay for long acting thyroid-stimulating (LATS) I went to the United States in 1970 as a trainee Fellow at the Johns Hopkins Hospital in Baltimore in Nuclear Medicine. Johns Hopkins Nuclear Medicine under Henry Wagner was regarded at that time as the leading training centre for nuclear medicine worldwide. After spending 2 years there and gaining the American Boards in Nuclear Medicine I returned in 1972 to be appointed consultant in Nuclear Medicine at Guy's Hospital to establish the first nuclear medicine department in that hospital.

After 12 years in this post he was appointed Professor of Radiological Sciences with a remit to organise undergraduate and postgraduate teaching and research in diagnostic imaging into one organisation with strong science base. A significant early achievement was to obtain the first high field strength MRI machine and to give opportunities for the skills and roles of non-medical scientists within the discipline. In 1992 the U.K.'s first clinical PET centre for diagnosis and research was established within the division of radiological sciences.

Amongst other things I was president of BNMS and later the British Institute of Radiology retiring in 2003.

Bone Radionuclide Imaging, Quantitation and Bone Densitometry

15

Glen M. Blake and Ignac Fogelman

15.1 Radionuclide Imaging of Bone

It was the development of the cyclotron by Ernest Lawrence at Berkeley during the 1930s that first made radionuclides available in the quantity and variety to allow investigations of their medical use. Lawrence's brother John, who was a physician, directed the first clinical studies, which included an investigation by Charles Pecher of the treatment of metastatic bone disease with ^{89}Sr [1]. An important finding made at Berkeley was the discovery of ^{99m}Tc in 1938 by Segrè and Seaborg in a sample of irradiated molybdenum [2]. But further developments had to await the end of the war.

Since calcium has no radioisotopes suitable for imaging, the next obvious element to exploit was strontium. In 1959 Bauer and Wendeberg [3] described the first clinical study with ^{85}Sr ($E\gamma = 514$ keV; $T_{1/2} = 65$ days), but its use was limited by the long half-life and consequent high radiation dose. In 1964 Charkes, Sklaroff and Bierly [4] described skeletal scintigraphy with ^{87m}Sr ($E\gamma = 388$ keV; $T_{1/2} = 2.8$ h), a short half-life isomeric radionuclide conveniently available from a generator. ^{87m}Sr was the bone agent used in Sheffield where one of us (GB) started work in 1972. Its disadvantage was the high renal tubular reabsorption of strontium, which combined with the short half-life led to indistinct images with a high soft tissue background (Fig. 15.1).

A much superior agent, ^{18}F-fluoride, was described by Blau, Nagler and Bender in 1962 [5], but its use required an onsite cyclotron which was available in very few centres. By the early 1970s the situation was ripe for the introduction of ^{99m}Tc labelled bone radiopharmaceuticals.

G.M. Blake (✉) • I. Fogelman
Department of Nuclear Medicine, Guy's Campus, King's College London, London SE1 9RT, UK

© The Author(s) 2016
R. McCready et al. (eds.), *A History of Radionuclide Studies in the UK: 50th Anniversary of the British Nuclear Medicine Society*,
DOI 10.1007/978-3-319-28624-2_15

111

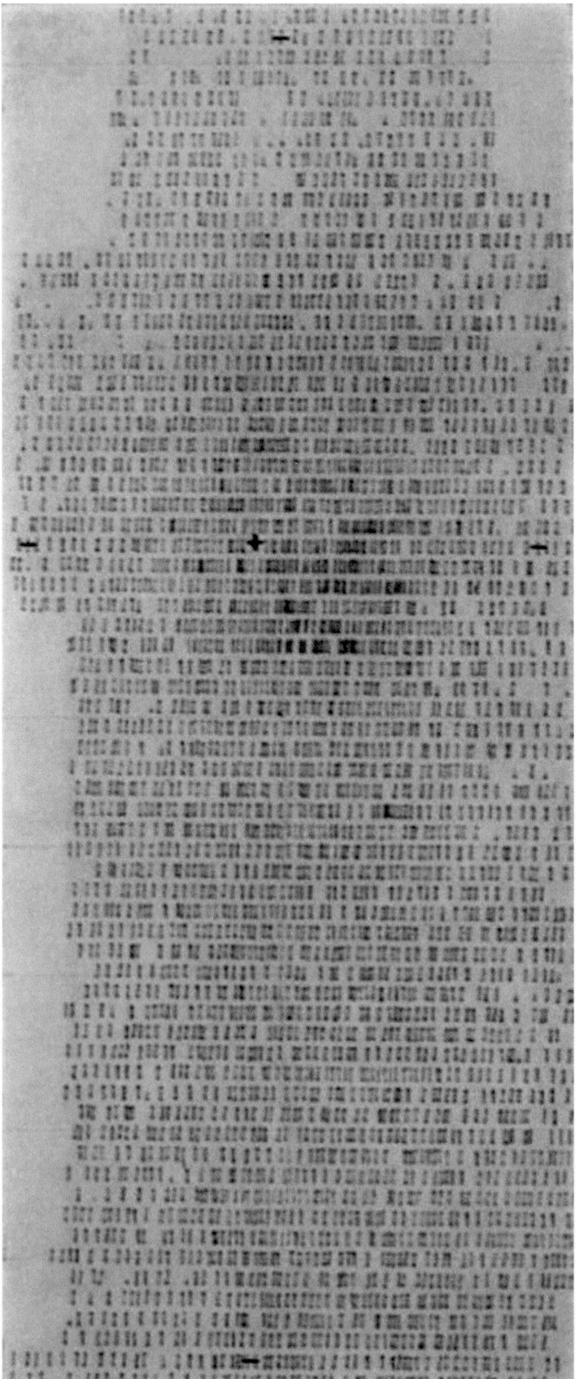

Fig. 15.1 Colour ribbon printout of an ^{87m}Sr bone scan performed on a rectilinear scanner (Reproduced with permission from Kemp et al. [20])

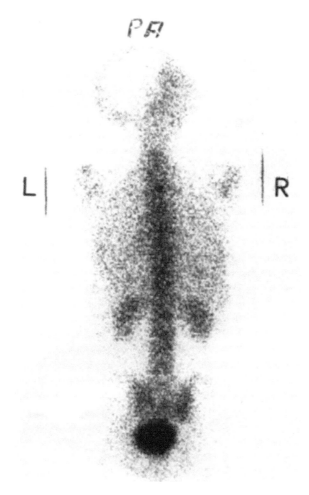

Fig. 15.2 Black and white film scintiscan from a rectilinear scanner showing a ^{99m}Tc-polyphosphate bone scan in a patient with no abnormalities (Reproduced with permission from Redman and Turley [21])

Interest in ^{99m}Tc for Nuclear Medicine imaging began in the early 1960s following the development of the ^{99m}Tc generator by Tucker and Greene at the Brookhaven laboratory [6]. The first technetium labelled bone agent, ^{99m}Tc-polyphosphate, was described by Subramanian and McAfee [7] in 1971 (Fig. 15.2), and so radical was the improvement in image quality that by 1973 ^{87m}Sr had fallen out of use.

In 1975 Subramanian described a superior agent, ^{99m}Tc-methylene diphosphonate [8], and with the introduction of the wide-field-of-view gamma camera and the replacement of spot views with whole-body scans the Nuclear Medicine bone scan took its modern form.

Recent years have seen a further change in the choice of optimum tracer as the wider availability of PET scanners has brought renewed interest in ^{18}F-fluoride. ^{18}F is superior to ^{99m}Tc-MDP for skeletal imaging because of its higher plasma clearance to bone and absence of protein binding, both factors that lead to improved bone to soft tissue uptake. In addition PET is a superior imaging technique with higher spatial resolution and sensitivity compared with the gamma camera. The ^{99m}Tc-MDP bone scan is an old and trusted friend that continues to perform with some distinction, but it is apparent that we can do significantly better with ^{18}F. As PET scanners become more widely available there appears to be a compelling case for the introduction of ^{18}F-fluoride as the preferred agent [9].

15.2   Quantitation of Bone Tracer Kinetics

There is a large early literature describing non-imaging studies of bone tracer kinetics using nuclides such as ^{45}Ca ($T_{1/2} = 163$ days), ^{47}Ca ($T_{1/2} = 4.5$ days) and ^{85}Sr ($T_{1/2} = 65$ days). Imaging studies using short half-life tracers such as ^{99m}Tc-MDP and ^{18}F-fluoride provide more restricted information, but have the advantage of allowing regional as well as whole skeleton measurements. Perhaps the most widely known bone quantitation method using an imaging tracer is the 24-h ^{99m}Tc-MDP whole-body retention test described by Fogelman in the late 1970s while working at the Glasgow Royal Infirmary [10]. In this test the patient is injected with a tracer amount (~1 MBq) of ^{99m}Tc-MDP and has a head-to-foot measurement in a shadow shield whole-body counter. The measurement is repeated 24 h later and, on the assumption the tracer is either cleared to bone or excreted through the kidneys, the counts are corrected for background and radioactive decay and the retention of ^{99m}Tc-MDP calculated. With the lack today of whole-body counter facilities, Brenner described a gamma camera measurement of whole-skeleton uptake based on whole-body scans acquired at 3 min and 6 h after injection [11]. By drawing a large region of interest over the adductor muscles the percentage of tracer still in soft tissue at 6 h is inferred and subtracted from the whole body retention to estimate the amount in bone.

A new method of using gamma camera scans to perform whole-skeleton and regional measurements of ^{99m}Tc-MDP bone plasma clearance (analogous to the measurement of renal function using GFR) was developed by Amelia Moore and colleagues at Guy's Hospital [12]. Fast (~10 min) anterior and posterior whole-body scans are performed at 10 min, 1, 2, 3 and 4 h after injection, and blood samples taken at 5, 20, 60, 120, 180 and 240 min. The latter are centrifuged by ultrafiltration to determine the plasma concentration of free (non-protein bound) ^{99m}Tc-MDP and the Patlak method used to determine whole-skeleton and regional (skull, spine, pelvis, arms, legs) bone plasma clearance. The method was used by Moore to investigate the effect of teriparatide on the bone scan in postmenopausal women treated for osteoporosis [13].

Just as PET imaging with ^{18}F-fluoride is superior to the ^{99m}Tc-MDP gamma camera scan, the same is true for bone quantitation. Hawkins et al. [14] described a method of measuring ^{18}F bone plasma clearance in the lumbar spine (units: mL min^{-1} mL^{-1}) by applying compartmental modelling to a 60-min dynamic PET scan with arterial sampling of the plasma curve. The method was simplified by Michelle Frost and colleagues at Guy's Hospital [15] so that from a series of venous blood samples and bed positions regional plasma clearance could be measured across the entire skeleton with a single injection of tracer. With the ability of ^{18}F PET scans to make measurements at the hip, the most important fracture site, we believe this is the best method for studying the effect of osteoporosis treatments on regional bone metabolism.

15.3   Bone Densitometry

The first bone densitometer based on photon absorptiometry was described by Cameron and Sorenson in 1963 [16] and used the 27 keV radiation from a ^{125}I source to measure bone mineral content in the radius, a method known as single photon absorptiometry (SPA). Because the beam contained photons with just a single energy it was necessary to place the patient's forearm in a water bath to simulate a constant thickness of soft tissue across the wrist.

During the 1970s Medical Physics groups at the University of Wisconsin and other centres pioneered the development of dual photon absorptiometry (DPA) using a rectilinear scanning device with a ^{153}Gd source with emissions at 44 and 100 keV [17]. Unlike SPA, these devices were able to scan the spine and hip. By the early 1980s several companies were manufacturing DPA scanners and in 1982 Frans Verlaan, founder of Vertec Scientific, organised a conference in London for those interested in the new technology that was attended by many from the Nuclear Medicine community. In some UK centres medical physicists such as Victor Poll in Southampton built their own systems from old rectilinear scanners. Because of the use of a radioactive source, the DPA devices were largely confined to Nuclear Medicine Departments with experience in the safe handling of radionuclides.

The limitation of DPA was that it is impossible to contain sufficient radioactivity in a small enough volume to achieve both the necessary count rate and adequate spatial resolution. In 1988 in the recently opened Guy's Osteoporosis Unit patient appointment times for the Novo BMC-LAB 22a DPA system were 1 h long, as it took 30 min to scan and analyse the spine, and a similar time for the hip (Fig. 15.3a, b).

In the same year bone densitometry was revolutionised when Jay Stein, founder of Hologic, replaced the ^{153}Gd source with an X-ray tube and produced the first dual-energy X-ray absorptiometry (DXA) system. This provided an improvement in scan quality for bone densitometry just as radical as ^{99m}Tc-MDP had for the radionuclide bone scan a decade earlier. Overnight the market for DPA systems was dead!

With a rapidly growing number of centres offering a DXA service it was necessary to devise clearer ways of reporting scans. In 1994 a group of physicians led by John Kanis recommended that DXA scans should be interpreted using T-scores defined as the BMD measurement expressed in standard deviation units relative to a population of healthy young adults, with osteoporosis defined as a T-score of less than −2.5 at the spine, hip or forearm [18]. This simple definition caught the imagination of clinicians and ever since the T-score has been a cornerstone of DXA scan reporting. But it ignores the fact that fracture risk increases progressively with

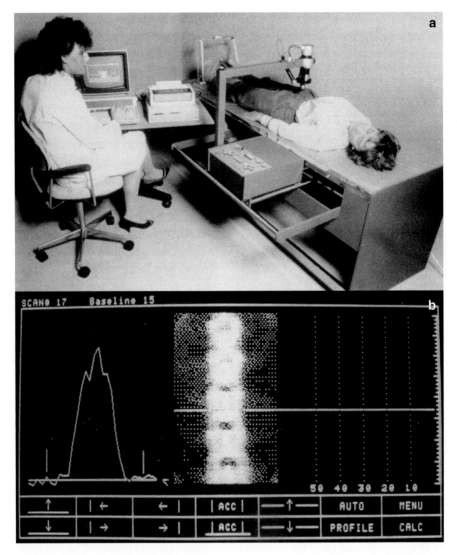

Fig. 15.3 (**a**) A Novo BMC-LAB 22a DPA scanner as used in the mid-1980s. (**b**) A lumbar spine DPA scan being analysed on a Novo BMC-LAB 22a system. Note the facility for the line-by-line adjustment of the soft tissue reference baseline on the left hand side of the image

diminishing BMD and does not take into account factors such as age and previous fractures in evaluating risk. In 2008 a collaboration under John Kanis placed the interpretation of DXA scans on a more secure footing by launching the FRAX website [19] where a clinician can enter details of a patient's hip T-score and clinical risk factors and obtain an estimate of their 10-year risk of fracture.

References

1. Pecher C. Biological investigations with radioactive calcium and strontium: preliminary report on the use of radioactive strontium in the treatment of metastatic bone cancer. Univ Calif Publ Pharmacol. 1942;2:117–49.
2. Segrè E, Seaborg GT. Nuclear isomerism in element 43. Phys Rev. 1938;54:772.
3. Bauer GC, Wendeberg B. External counting of Ca^{47} and Sr^{85} in studies of localised skeletal lesions in man. J Bone Joint Surg Br. 1959;41-B:558–80.
4. Charkes ND, Sklaroff DM, Bierly J. Detection of metastatic cancer to bone by scintiscanning with strontium-87 m. Am J Roentgenol Radium Ther Nucl Med. 1964;91:1121–7.
5. Blau M, Nagler W, Bender MA. Fluorine-18: a new isotope for bone scanning. J Nucl Med. 1962;3:332–4.
6. Richards P. Technetium-99m: the early days. 1989. Available at: http://www.osti.gov/scitech/servlets/purl/5612212/. Accessed 3 Sept 2015.
7. Subramanian G, McAfee JG. A new complex of ^{99m}Tc for skeletal imaging. Radiology. 1971;99:192–6.
8. Subramanian G, McAfee JG, Blair RJ, Kallfelz FA, Thomas FD. Technetium-99m-methylene diphosphonate - a superior agent for skeletal imaging: comparison with other technetium complexes. J Nucl Med. 1975;16:744–55.
9. Fogelman I, Blake GM, Cook GJ. The isotope bone scan: we can do better. Eur J Nucl Med Mol Imaging. 2013;40:1139–40.
10. Fogelman I, Bessent RG, Turner JG, Citrin DL, Boyle IT, Greig WR. The use of whole-body retention of Tc-99m diphosphonate in the diagnosis of metabolic bone disease. J Nucl Med. 1978;19:270–5.
11. Brenner W, Bohuslavizki KH, Sieweke N, Tinnemeyer S, Clausen M, Henze E. Quantification of diphosphonate uptake based on conventional bone scanning. Eur J Nucl Med. 1997;24:1284–90.
12. Moore AE, Blake GM, Fogelman I. Quantitative measurements of bone remodeling using ^{99m}Tc-methylene diphosphonate bone scans and blood sampling. J Nucl Med. 2008;49:375–82.
13. Moore AE, Blake GM, Taylor KA, Ruff VA, Rana AE, Wan X, Fogelman I. Changes observed in radionuclide bone scans during and after teriparatide treatment for osteoporosis. Eur J Nucl Med Mol Imaging. 2012;39:326–36.
14. Hawkins RA, Choi Y, Huang SC, Hoh CK, Dahlbom M, Schiepers C, Satyamurthy N, Barrio JR, Phelps ME. Evaluation of the skeletal kinetics of fluorine-18-fluoride ion with PET. J Nucl Med. 1992;33:633–42.
15. Frost ML, Moore AE, Siddique M, Blake GM, Laurent D, Borah B, Schramm U, Valentin MA, Pellas TC, Marsden PK, Schleyer PJ, Fogelman I. ^{18}F-fluoride PET as a noninvasive imaging biomarker for determining treatment efficacy of bone active agents at the hip: a prospective, randomized, controlled clinical study. J Bone Miner Res. 2013;28:1337–47.
16. Cameron JR, Sorenson J. Measurement of bone mineral in vivo: an improved method. Science. 1963;142:230–2.

17. Wilson CR, Madsen M. Dichromatic absorptiometry of vertebral bone mineral content. Invest Radiol. 1977;12:180–4.
18. WHO technical report series 843: assessment of fracture risk and its application to screening for postmenopausal osteoporosis. Geneva: World Health Organization; 1994.
19. World Health Organization Collaborating Centre for Metabolic Bone Diseases. FRAX® WHO fracture risk assessment tool web version 3.9, released 17 Oct 2014. Available at: http://www.shef.ac.uk/FRAX. Accessed 3 Sept 2015.
20. Kemp HBS, Johns DL, McAlister J, Goodlee JN. The role of fluorine-18 and strontium-87m scintigraphy in the management of infective spondylitis. J Bone Joint Surg. 1973;55:301–11.
21. Redman JF, Turley JT. Technetium polyphosphate bone scans in carcinoma of the prostate. Urology. 1973;1:218–20.

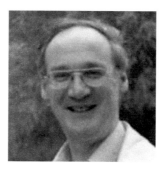

Glen M. Blake I was born in Walthamstow in East London and was fortunate to benefit from the 11-Plus exam, going to Chigwell School in Essex. I won an open scholarship to study Physics at Oxford and came out with the top first in my year group. After that I did a PhD in the Radio Astronomy group at the Cavendish Laboratory under Martin Ryle. My interest in Medical Physics developed from a fellow research student, Lawrence Oldfield, who had just returned from a year working in Canada in radiotherapy. My first post in the NHS was in Sheffield where the Medical Physics Department was led by Harold Miller. Harold had been a student of James Chadwick in 1932, the year that Chadwick discovered the neutron. I worked in the Isotope Unit at the Sheffield Royal Infirmary, and later at the Hallamshire Hospital when it opened in 1978. There I worked with John Kanis on a grant proposal to purchase one of the early DPA bone density scanners for research projects in Sheffield. In 1984 I moved to the Nuclear Medicine Department at Southampton under Duncan Ackery where I widened my experience and was involved with projects that included the use of ^{89}Sr to treat metastatic bone disease. In 1989 I moved to the Nuclear Medicine Department at Guy's Hospital under Ignac Fogelman. Here I had the opportunity to take up bone densitometry again in the recently opened Osteoporosis Unit. At Guy's I became more heavily involved with teaching and supervising research students, and in 2003 I moved from the NHS to work for King's College London, becoming Professor of Osteoporosis in 2012.

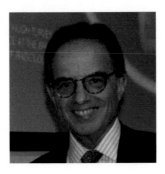

Ignac Fogelman Professor Ignac Fogelman is currently Professor of Nuclear Medicine at King's College London and Honorary Consultant Physician at Guy's and St Thomas' NHS Trust and Director of the Osteoporosis Screening and Research Unit, Guy's Hospital. Professor Fogelman did his medical training in the Professorial Department of Medicine at the Glasgow Royal Infirmary where he developed his interest in metabolic bone disease working with Dr Iain Boyle and Dr Rodney Bessent. At that time Nuclear Medicine in Glasgow came under the wing of the Department of Medicine, and the newly available ^{99m}Tc-diphosphonate imaging agents proved a useful means of investigating metabolic bone disease, leading to the first of over 400 publications and the completion of his MD. His appointment as Consultant Physician in the Nuclear Medicine Department at Guy's Hospital in 1983 gave further opportunities to develop his interests in bone. In 1988 he instigated the first osteoporosis screening service in the UK, initially using a DPA scanner and later one of the first DXA systems. In 1996 he became Professor of Nuclear Medicine. He has written or edited 15 books and supervised 17 PhD/MD students. He is a former board member and trustee of the National Osteoporosis Society and was previously chairman of its Bone Densitometry Forum. Professor Fogelman is currently chairman of the board of examiners for the MSc in Nuclear Medicine at King's College, which provides the only recognised training programme for Nuclear Medicine in the UK.

Therapeutic Nuclear Medicine in the UK

16

John Buscombe

16.1 Introduction

Therapeutic Nuclear Medicine in the United Kingdom has developed in a fairly inconsistent way over the last 50 years. It is a sad inditement of the state of British nuclear medicine that access to good therapeutic nuclear medicine has become little more than a "post code lottery" [1]. This in part has been due to the uneven spread of specialists in nuclear medicine with most posts being concentrated in the South East and North West. It is not therefore surprising that most therapeutic nuclear medicine has developed in these areas as well. Diagnostic nuclear medicine was traditionally performed by nuclear medicine physicians and radiologists but the latter have generally showed little interest in radionuclide therapy as it was not seen as "radiology". An alternate source of expertise lies with clinical oncology and in many parts of the U.K radionuclide therapy is delivered by clinical oncologists. However, as oncologists have taken a system based approach to treatment and those who are licenced to treat thyroid cancer may have little interest in cancers in other sites. Compounded to this has been decision by clinical oncologists to withdraw from treatment of benign disease. Some endocrinologists have taken on the role of treating benign thyroid disease but of course they will not do radiation synevectomies. The delivery of radionuclide therapy also requires further craft group skills in particular trained clinical scientists, technologists, radiopharmacy and nursing. All this has led to a centripetal effect with expertise being concentrated in less than ten centres across the UK. The majority of these centres lie within Greater London further exacerbating the poor geographic distribution of services. The biggest change over the past 5 years which may be temporary change in funding with

J. Buscombe
Department of Nuclear Medicine, Cambridge University Hospitals,
Cambridge CB2 0QQ, UK

© The Author(s) 2016
R. McCready et al. (eds.), *A History of Radionuclide Studies in the UK:
50th Anniversary of the British Nuclear Medicine Society*,
DOI 10.1007/978-3-319-28624-2_16

central funding in England for radium-223, peptide radionuclide radiotherapy (PRRT) and to a lesser extent yttrium-90 particulates for selective intra-arterial radio-therapy (SIRT) for metastasis in the liver. For those centres who already offer a range of radionuclide therapies adding these newer treatments has some resource implications but does not normally require extensive business planning to get approval to start treatments. Therefore even with new funding patients have tended to be seen and treated in those centres who have already undertaken a range of radionuclide therapies.

16.2 Radioiodine

The greatest success story for radionuclide therapy has been the use of I-131 for both benign and malignant thyroidal disease [2]. Since the first treatments 70 years ago in Manchester most patients in the United Kingdom have access to I-131 and the specialist clinics that have been developed for assessing the need for treatment and follow-up. In benign thyroid disease it has been shown that early treatment with I-131 is cost effective and preferable to years of trials of anti-thyroid medication. It is considered routine (Fig. 16.1) but once was a revolution, quoting the great Ralston Paterson from Manchester "The first point to be emphasised is that this use of radio-iodine in thyroid cancer represents a completely new principle of therapy—the principle of systemic ingestion with, thereafter, selective absorption of a drug carrying

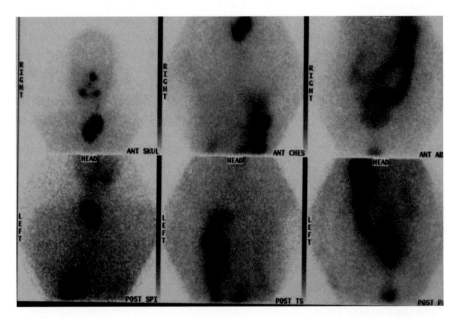

Fig. 16.1 A series of spot gamma camera images from the 1980s showing residual uptake in the neck and physiological activity in the large bowel

a radioactive element in it and resulting in a zone of localised high radiation dosage in the selective absorption tissues".

Once thought too dangerous to give to young women it would now be considered ideal especially if they were considering having children. In thyroid cancer, there has been a rare British triumph with the recent "HiLo" trial showing that for those with low risk cancers ablation with 1.1 GBq is as good as using 3.7 GBq [3]. This has resulted in a reduction in the risk of radioiodine associated morbidity and of much greater interest to the managers of the National Health Service a reduced number of days in a hospital bed.

16.3 Relieving Bone Pain

The second theme in radionuclide therapy was the relief of bone pain. Initially this depended on the use of phosphorus-32 a bone seeking radiopharmaceutical. However, its long half-life resulted in a high level of bone marrow suppression. The next strategy was to administer a radiopharmaceutical to an area of limited disease and thus radiation synovectomy was developed with an emphasis of Y-90 colloids injected into inflamed knees. A technique which consistently delivers pain relief in 80 % of patients to whom it is administered with relief of pain lasting 12 months or more. However, the number of practitioners who regularly give this safe and inexpensive treatments are so rare that when the author had a private practice in Harley Street, good business was had by flying patients over from New York for treatment.

Then came another British story. There remained great need for a radionuclide that could treat the pain from bone metastases but not have the side effects of P-32. Looking down the periodic table below calcium lies strontium and Sr-89 could deliver a soft beta with a short path length but still a long half-life. This product was developed by the newly privatised Amersham International with Prof Duncan Ackery from Southampton [4], his clinical scientist Dr Glenn Blake and two registrars Sandy McEwan and Val Lewington. The science was great as 70 % of patients had good or complete pain relief, the marketing was abysmal. The American Merrell-Dow company developed a Samarium diphosphonate (Sm-153 EDTMP) as a sort of strontium "light" with a shorter half-life it could be used in those with higher disease burdens [5]. This was the first radionuclide therapy in which a full phase III clinical trial was performed but after looking like it would be a success interest also fizzled out after a decade.

The latest incarnation is another group-2 element Radium-223 which has been jointly developed by Bayer and the Norwegian company Algeta. After a clinical trial of 1000 patients (the largest contributing country being the UK) it was shown that 6 cycles of Ra-223 not only reduced the pain from bone metastases of prostate cancer but patients lived longer [6]. Therefore with Ra-223 patients liver better and liver longer. So far Ra-223 looks to be successful but time will tell.

16.4 Theranostics

Though the term theranostics is relatively recent, nuclear medicine has been performing theranostics since the first radioiodine scan. The meaning of the word theranostics is not clearly defined but is generally understood to mean combining relevant diagnostic and therapeutic methods. This is ideally suited to nuclear medicine and the first designed theranostic agent was first used in the United Kingdom in 1986 by the Southampton group using low activity I-131 meta-iodo benzyl guinadine (MIBG) and then high activity I-131 MIBG to treat malignant phaeochromocytomas [7] and later its use was expanded into other tumour types such as carcinoid [8] and more importantly neuroblastoma with much work being done at University College Hospital London (UCHL) by Drs Jamshed Bomanji and Dr Mark Gaze.

The most successful form of theranostics however, has been the use of somatostatin analogues for the treatment of neuroendocrine tumours. This method was first proposed by Prof Eric Krenning in Rotterdam [9] but using various methods has become more widely used in the United Kingdom with many centres using the optimised imaging of Ga-68 DOTATATE PET and Lu-177 DOTATATE therapy. Though not licenced products these agents hold European Medicine Agency orphan drug status. Also presently those patients being treated for disseminated neuroendocrine tumours which are resistant to chemotherapy or biologicals can have the radioactive treatment funded centrally within England. Using this approach it looks as though 70–80 % of patients have a good palliative outcome with a low rate (1–4 %) of significant long lasting toxicity [10].

However not all theranostic agents have proved to be so accepted Y-90 tostisuomab is an antibody that can be used to treat CD20 expressing non-Hodgkins lymphomas (NHL). However, despite clear evidence that a single treatment can be as effective as several months of biologicals [11] it has failed to be used widely and must be considered a commercial failure. The reasons for this failure is unclear but it had to compete with other non-radioactive agents supported by large pharmaceutical companies with large advertising budgets.

It seems that theranostic radionuclide therapy will only be allowed to be successful where it does not threaten the commercial interest of large organisations but in reality this still gives us many rarer tumours, which often have unique targets, which we can aim to treat.

16.5 The Double-Whammy

The basis of most radionuclide therapy has been the systemic administration of a product that will use a molecular target such as a somatostatin receptor and this was the principle laid out by Paterson in 1950. However, what if the target disease is limited to one organ, would it not be possible to direct a treatment to that one organ and maximise the radioactivity delivered and reduce the radioactive dose to other tissues. Since the earliest days of nuclear medicine there have been attempts to do this for example giving I-131 lipiodol into the leg lymphatics of a patient with

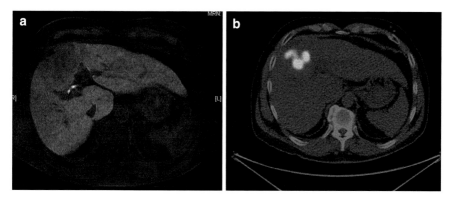

Fig. 16.2 (**a**) A LAVA MR sequence showing a large primary HCC in segment 4. (**b**) A Y-90 Time of flight PET showing precise delivery of Y-90 resin particulates into segment 4 and localisation in the tumour delivering over 150 Gy tumour dose with minimal radiation to the rest of the liver

lymphoma or instilling Y-90 into the peritoneal cavity [12, 13]. The breakthrough came with the advances of a different technology; that of fast low dose fluoroscopy and interventional catheter design.

The liver would be a good target, there is no doubt that primary and secondary tumours in the liver are unlikely to be result in a long and happy life. The liver has a twin arterial blood supply but uniquely primary and secondary liver tumours are fed by the hepatic artery but normal hepatocytes also has an additional blood supply via the portal vein. A catheter placed in the relevant hepatic artery will deliver a radioactive substance which may have a radiation and an embolic effect so the tumour gets a "double whammy".

This idea was first used in a reasonable number of patients in Rennes in France using I-131 Lipiodol in primary hepatocellular cancer and brought to the UK by Dr Andrew Hilson at the Royal Free Hospital where it was shown to be as effective as chemotherapy loaded lipiodol but with fewer side effects [14, 15].

The next major steps took place in Canada with Y-90 labelled glass beads (Theraspheres) and in Australia Y-90 labelled resin beads (SIRspheres). In Clinical trials the use of these products in patients with metastases from colon cancer has been shown to improve survival [16]. Their use in the UK was pioneered in London by Prof Al-Nahhas at the Hammersmith Hospital and Dr Buxton-Thomas in Kings College Hospital. Presently their use is funded in 12 sites around England for evaluation by the radiotherapy clinical reference group in metastatic colo-rectal cancer but probably their greatest potential use to save lives is with hepatocelluar cancer (Fig. 16.2) but it is in this disease these treatments remain unfunded by the National Health Service.

16.6 Dosimetry

One area of deficiency in radionuclide therapy has been in the field of dosimetry. With external beam radiotherapy the distribution of radioactivity is highly predictable. This is not the case with systemic radionuclide therapy. Post therapy imaging is needed to look for the biodistribution of agents. However, an inherent problem is that molecular agents may not distribute homogeneously within a target tissue and these subtle changes may not be picked up by a technique which has a resolution of 1–2 cm. In addition there are no agreed methodologies for calculating radiation doses or even what doses to calculate. It may be fairly easy to measure the whole body radioactivity every day in a patient who has received I-131 but how does that translate to a radiation dose to the salivary glands or even the target tumour?

If dosimetry is to be done and it is a legal requirement it is done there should be consensus on how dosimetry is done and what methods are used. In health systems that are becoming increasing short of resources it is vital that the radionuclide therapy community identify what personnel and training is needed to deliver dosimetry of high quality to all sites using these treatments [1].

16.7   The Future

When the BNMS celebrates its 75th anniversary will there be a chapter on radionuclide therapy? This is difficult to know. Many of us passionately believe in these methods but we have to accept that even in the nuclear medicine community we are a minority.

The recent appointment of Val Lewington as the UK's first professor of Nuclear Medicine with a special interest in radionuclide therapy must be a step in the right direction, however there is much to do. Radionuclide therapy is integral to the nuclear medicine curriculum but how many trainees really get to be immersed in therapy-still too few I fear.

As we enter into the age of personalized medicine theranostics and radionuclide therapy should become more important not less. This however, will need investment on a scale not seen before and a cadre of trained and enthusiastic nuclear medicine practitioners from all craft groups.

References

1. Flux G, Moss L, Buscombe J, Gaze M, Guy M, Mather S, Orchard K. Molecular radiotherapy in the UK. London: British Institute of Radiology; 2011.
2. Paterson R. The treatment of thyroid carcinoma with radioiodine. Br J Radiol. 1950;23:553–6.

3. Mallick U, Harmer C, Yap B, et al. Ablation with low dose radioiodine and thyrotropin alfa in thyroid cancer. N Engl J Med. 2012;366:1674–85.
4. Lewington VJ, McEwan AJ, Ackery DM, et al. A prospective randomised double blind cross-over study to examine the efficacy of strontium-89 in pain palliation in patients with advanced prostate cancer metastatic to bone. Eur J Cancer. 1991;27:954–8.
5. Serafini AN, Houston SJ, Resche I, et al. Palliation of pain associated with metastatic bone pain using samarium-153 lexidronam: a double blind placebo controlled clinical trial. J Clin Oncol. 1998;16:1574–81.
6. Parker C, Nilsson S, Heinrich D, et al. Alpha emitter radium-223 and survival in metastatic prostate cancer. N Engl J Med. 2013;369:213–23.
7. McEwan AJ, Shapiro B, Sisson JC, Beierwaltes WH, Ackery DM. Radio-iodobenzylguanadine for the scintigraphic location and therapy of adrenergic tumours. Semin Nucl Med. 1985;15:132–5.
8. Prvulovich EM, Stein RC, Bomanji JB, Ledermann JA, Taylor I, Ell PJ. Iodine-131 MIBG therapy of a patient with carcinoid liver metastases. J Nucl Med. 1998;39:1743–5.
9. Krenning EP, Kooij PP, Bakker WH, et al. Radiotherapy with a radiolabeled somatostain analogue [111In-DTPA-D-Phe1]-octreotide. A case history. Ann N Y Acad Sci. 1994;733:496–506.
10. Buscombe J, Navalkissoor S. Molecualr radiotherapy. Clin Med. 2012;12:381–6.
11. Witzig TE, Molina A, Gordon LI, et al. Long term responses in patients with recurring or refractory B cell non-Hodgkin lymphoma treated with yttrium-90 ibritumomab tiuxetan. Cancer. 2007;109;1804–10.
12. Hiniakowa I, Skalska-Vorbrodt J. Intralymphatic treatment of various neoplasms with radio-isotope I-131. Clinical considerations. Pol Przegl Radiol Med Nukl. 1971;35:83–90.
13. Heneghan JB, Crook JN, Cohn I. Yttrium-90 microspheres for inhibition of intra-peritoneal tumor growth. Surg Forum. 1968;19:78–80.
14. Bretagne JF, Raul JL, Bourguet P, et al. Hepatic artery injection of I-131 labelled lipiodol. Part II. Preliminary results of therapeutic use in patients with hepatocellular carcinoma and liver metastases. Radiology. 1988;162:547–50.
15. Bhattacharya S, Novell JR, Dusciko GM, Hison AJ, Dick R, Hobbs KE. Epirubacin-Lipiodol chemotherapy versus 131- iodine-Lipiodol in the treatment of unresectable hepatocellular cancer. Cancer. 1995;76:2202–10.
16. Gray B, Van Hazel G, Hope M, Burton M, Moroz P, Anderson J, Gebski V. Randomised trial of SIR-spheres plus chemotherapy vs chemotherapy alone for treating patients with liver metastases from primary bowel cancer. Ann Oncol. 2001;12:1711–20.

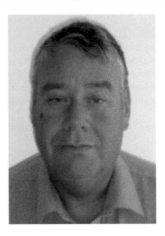

John Buscombe I trained in general internal medicine in London and Essex before being trained in Nuclear Medicine at the Middlesex Hospital, London.

My first Consultant post was at the Royal Free Hospital in London, I developed one of Europe's busiest therapeutic nuclear medicine practices. This included the development of directly inject-able radiopharmaceuticals into arteries supplying brain and liver tumours. During this time, I was involved in a range of research projects including Phase I and II trials in both diagnostic and thera-peutic nuclear medicine and also acted as principal investigator in international Phase III trials. These trials included the use of 99mTc MIBI in identifying and risk stratifying breast cancer and agents for imaging lung cancer and pulmonary emboli as well as the use of radioimmunotherapy for colon cancer and Hodgkin's lymphoma.

Since 2010 I have been working at Cambridge University Hospitals with a particular emphasis in cyclotron-based PET. The focus of these projects has been on the use of C-11 products in iden-tifying sub-centimetre endocrine tumours and also PET imaging of atheroma and cardiovascular inflammation. I am also a Professor of Nuclear Medicine in the University of Pretoria developing nuclear medicine and education in an African setting

I have published over 200 papers in peer-reviewed journals, written or edited s7 books and written over 40 book chapters. I continue to work for the nuclear medicine community in the UK and Europe and have been a Council Member for the British Nuclear Medicine Society twice and has also served on the British Nuclear Medicine Society annual meeting scientific committee for a total of 6 years.

Hospital Radiopharmacy in the UK

17

James R. Ballinger

The first great expansion in nuclear medicine took place around 1970 with the introduction of the ^{99}Mo/^{99m}Tc generator and kit preparations, allowing convenient on site production of radiopharmaceuticals. That being said, I would be remiss if I did not begin by mentioning the seminal work of Stephen Garnett (much later my PhD supervisor) in development of the ^{51}Cr EDTA technique for determination of glomerular filtration rate [1].

In the early days, hospital radiopharmacy usually fell under the remit of medical physics and regulation was somewhat informal. The Medicines Act 1968 was the first legislation to classify radiopharmaceuticals as drugs. In the early 1970s, the Medicines Control Agency (MCA, later Medicines and Healthcare Products Regulatory Agency, MHRA) took an interest in improving the standards for practice of radiopharmacy but at this point theirs was only an advisory role. An early guideline on preparation of radiopharmaceuticals in hospitals was published by the British Institute of Radiology in 1975 [2]. With the loss of Crown Immunity in 1991, radiopharmacy came under the full scrutiny of the MHRA and standards have been continually tightened since then. Indeed, the UK led the world in this, for which the world does not thank us.

Hospital radiopharmacy is now one of the most heavily regulated specialties imaginable. Radiopharmaceuticals are drugs (MHRA) but also radioactive materials (Environment Agency), sources of radioactive exposure (Health and Safety Executive), for which patient exposure must be optimized (Care Quality Commission) and which must be transported safely (Office of Nuclear Regulation). Moreover, these different regulatory agencies can have conflicting requirements. For safety of the operator, radioactive materials should be handled under negative

J.R. Ballinger
Imaging Sciences, King's College London, London, UK

© The Author(s) 2016
R. McCready et al. (eds.), *A History of Radionuclide Studies in the UK:
50th Anniversary of the British Nuclear Medicine Society*,
DOI 10.1007/978-3-319-28624-2_17

129

air pressure but for safety of the patient these procedures should be under positive pressure. For safety of the operator in case of contamination there should be a sink nearby, but sterile pharmaceuticals must not be handled anywhere near a sink. One issue they all agree on is that disposable gloves and gowns are a good idea. As such a specialist area, few of the agency inspectors have full understanding, which can lead to disastrous outcomes. A classic case occurred some 15 years ago when an MHRA inspector insisted that a radiopharmacy sanitise its kits with chlorine based disinfectants rather than the usual alcohol; the next day all the products failed because ^{99m}Tc labeling requires reducing conditions but the residual chlorine was an oxidant.

It is believed that the first hospital radiopharmacy in the UK was established at the Liverpool Clinic in the late 1950s. Most radiopharmacies at major teaching hospitals were set up in the early 1970s. Radiopharmacy as a specialty became recognized under the Regional Pharmacists Committee and the first formal meeting of radiopharmacists took place on 26 January 1977 at a pub in Cambridgeshire. In attendance were Malcolm Frier (Nottingham General Hospital), Stuart Hesslewood (City Hospital, Birmingham), Penny Hill (Bristol Royal Infirmary), Colin Lazarus (Guy's Hospital, London), Bill Little (Royal Liverpool Hospital), and Teresa McCarthy (Addenbrooke's Hospital, Cambridge). The Regional Radiopharmacists Subcommittee eventually morphed into the UK Radiopharmacy Group (UKRG) under which name it is still going strong (www.ukrg.org.uk). UKRG remains a public sector organisation (there are no commercial members) with broadly geographical representation and includes members from PET, IPEM, MHRA, and academia.

Since the 1990s the UKRG has held an annual workshop open to the radiopharmacy community and industry in January at The Beeches conference centre in Bourneville, Birmingham. Attendance has grown to about sixty, the capacity of the venue. In the mid 1990s, UKRG published the UK Radiopharmacy Handbook, which was updated in 2002. Much of the content in the original handbook is now easily accessible via the internet, but certain sections remain on the UKRG website as Radiopharmacy Information Resources. UKRG has also published guidance documents on a variety of issues.

Also since the 1990s an annual postgraduate lecture course in radiopharmacy has been held at King's College London under the auspices of the UKRG. Originally set up by Tony Theobald (KCL) and Stephen Mather (St Bartholomew's Hospital, Queen Mary University, Cancer Research Campaign), it has latterly been organised by Jim Ballinger (KCL, Guy's and St Thomas' Hospital). This is open to anyone interested in the field and is offered for credit to students on the MSc in Nuclear Medicine Science (KCL), MSc in Pharmaceutical Technology and Quality Assurance (PTQA; originally at the University of Leeds, now at University of Manchester), and the new MSc in Clinical Pharmaceutical Science (University of Manchester). Annual attendance varies between 20 and 45. UKRG has also co-sponsors with KCL a biannual practical course in radiochemical purity testing; laboratory space limits attendance to 20.

The UKRG has maintained a database of adverse reactions and product defects. For many years annual summaries were published in the European Journal of Nuclear Medicine blue pages and the plan is for this tradition to resume.

Throughout the years, UKRG members have played an important role in such UK organisations as the British Nuclear Medicine Society (BNMS) and the Administration of Radioactive Substances Advisory Committee (ARSAC), as well as the European Association of Nuclear Medicine (EANM). The biannual European Symposium on Radiopharmacy and Radiopharmaceuticals has been hosted in the UK on three occasions.

Charles Sampson (Addenbrooke's Hospital, Cambridge) edited the Textbook of Radiopharmacy in 1990. It is now in its fourth edition, edited by Tony Theobald, and renamed Sampson's Textbook of Radiopharmacy in Charlie's honour.

There have been many developments in Positron Emission Tomography (PET) in which the UK has played a major role, with the original two PET centres at the Hammersmith Hospital and the University of Aberdeen, and the first clinical PET centre at Guy's and St Thomas' Hospital. However, this development has largely been in parallel with hospital radiopharmacy rather than part of it; both fields have been poorer because of this missed opportunity.

The presence in the UK of one of the largest radiopharmaceutical companies, Amersham International, now part of GE Healthcare, meant that a number of new ^{99m}Tc labeled radiopharmaceuticals were first put into humans in UK nuclear medicine departments. These include cerebral perfusion imaging with ^{99m}Tc HMPAO (Ceretec) at the Middlesex Hospital [3] and Aberdeen [4], myocardial perfusion imaging with ^{99m}Tc tetrofosmin (Myoview), based on chemistry developed at the University of Cardiff, also at Aberdeen [5], and hypoxia imaging with ^{99m}Tc HL91 (Prognox, never marketed) at Guy's Hospital [6]. Mention must also be made of the development of cell radiolabeling techniques by the group under the direction of Michael Peters at the Hammersmith Hospital, leading to ^{111}In tropolonate [7] and ^{99m}Tc HMPAO [8] becoming standard labeling methods worldwide. This is now being extended to subpopulations of cells [9]. Over the last 50 years we have witnessed great changes within the radiopharmaceutical industry, as I have chronicled elsewhere [10]. At times the radiopharmaceutical divisions have suffered as minor cogs in the big wheel of a pharmaceutical or chemical company.

Within pharmacy, radiopharmacy has suffered by being classified as a technical service when in reality it is among the most clinical of specialties. The radiopharmacy is often embedded in a clinical nuclear medicine department where it is impossible to avoid patients even if one wanted to. Where else can one see the full gamut — from raw materials to injectable product to clinical results — all within a matter of minutes to hours? I'm still amazed every time I see a beating heart on the processing monitor. But pharmacy is only one route into radiopharmacy, and the lack of a defined career path has created problems in recruitment and succession planning. Finally in 2013 Health Education England set up a scientist training programme in Clinical Pharmaceutical Science which will lead to state registration with the Health and Caring Professions Council (HCPC). Finally, formal recognition of radiopharmacy.

In summary, the practice of hospital radiopharmacy has become much more tightly controlled over the last 50 years. Ensuring high standards has been expensive both in terms of operating and capital costs. Ironically, this has protected NHS radiopharmacies by making the UK unattractive for commercial radiopharmacies. But this has also slowed the implementation of new procedures which are virtually routine elsewhere; witness the limited availability of ^{68}Ga labeled peptides in the UK. My greatest sadness is that the diversion of human resources to regulatory issues has virtually killed hospital based radiopharmaceutical research and development in the UK. Despite this, members of the UK community continue to play an important role nationally and internationally in advancing the practice of hospital radiopharmacy.

References

1. Garnett ES, Parsons V, Veall N. Measurement of glomerular filtration-rate in man using a ^{51}Cr-edetic-acid complex. Lancet. 1967;1:818–9.
2. Taylor DM, Brock M, Frier M, Joshi VK, Jewkes R, Keeling DH, Hughes D, Little WA, Smith PH, Trott NG, Watson IA, Whately TL, Wood EJ. Guidelines for the preparation of radiopharmaceuticals in hospitals. London: British Institute of Radiology; 1975.
3. Ell PJ, Jarritt PH, Cullum I, Hocknell JM, Costa DC, Lui D, Jewkes RF, Steiner TJ, Nowotnik DP, Pickett RD, et al. Regular cerebral blood flow mapping with ^{99m}Tc-labelled compound. Lancet. 1985;2:50–1.
4. Sharp PF, Smith FW, Gemmell HG, Lyall D, Evans NT, Gvozdanovic D, Davidson J, Tyrrell DA, Pickett RD, Neirinckx RD. Technetium-99m HM-PAO stereoisomers as potential agents for imaging regional cerebral blood flow: human volunteer studies. J Nucl Med. 1986;27: 171–7.
5. Higley B, Smith FW, Smith T, Gemmell HG, Das Gupta P, Gvozdanovic DV, Graham D, Hinge D, Davidson J, Lahiri A. Technetium-99m-1,2-bis[bis(2-ethoxyethyl)-phosphino]ethane: human biodistribution, dosimetry and safety of a new myocardial perfusion imaging agent. J Nucl Med. 1993;34:30–8.
6. Cook GJ, Houston S, Barrington SF, Fogelman I. Technetium-99m-labeled HL91 to identify tumor hypoxia: correlation with fluorine-18-FDG. J Nucl Med. 1998;39:99–103.
7. Peters AM, Saverymuttu SH, Reavy HJ, Danpure HJ, Osman S, Lavender JP. Imaging of inflammation with indium-111 tropolonate labeled leukocytes. J Nucl Med. 1983;24: 39–44.
8. Peters AM, Danpure HJ, Osman S, Hawker RJ, Henderson BL, Hodgson HJ, Kelly JD, Neirinckx RD, Lavender JP. Clinical experience with ^{99m}Tc-hexamethylpropylene-amineoxime for labelling leucocytes and imaging inflammation. Lancet. 1986;2:946–9.

9. Lukawska JJ, Livieratos L, Sawyer BM, Lee T, O'Doherty M, Blower PJ, Kofi M, Ballinger JR, Corrigan CJ, Gnanasegaran G, Sharif-Paghaleh E, Mullen GE. Real-time differential tracking of human neutrophil and eosinophil migration in vivo. J Allergy Clin Immunol. 2014;133:233–9.
10. Ballinger J. News and views. Nucl Med Commun. 2014;35:218–20.

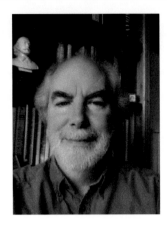

James R. Ballinger I retired in 2015 after spending 31 years in clinical radiopharmacy, half of that time in Canada, the remainder in the UK. Born in Toronto, I obtained my BSc in Pharmacy from the University of Toronto in 1976, followed by an MSc in analytical toxicology. I was then persuaded to undertake a 1-year residency in radiopharmacy at Chedoke-McMaster Hospital in Hamilton, followed by a PhD in PET radiochemistry, where my project involved synthesis and evaluation of ^{18}F-fluoronicotine for regional cerebral perfusion studies and investigation of the nicotinic acetylcholine receptor. In 1984 I took a position as radiopharmacist at Ottawa Civic Hospital where I developed a profile as an independent researcher. I moved to the Ontario Cancer Institute and Princess Margaret Hospital in Toronto in 1990 and continued research in multidrug resistance to chemotherapy and hypoxia imaging. In 1999, perhaps unwisely, I migrated against the rotation of the earth to take a post at Addenbrooke's Hospital in Cambridge. My final move was in 2003 to Guy's and St Thomas' Hospital and King's College London, where I was involved in setting up and teaching on the MSc in Radiopharmaceutics and PET Radiochemistry. I am a fellow of the Royal Society of Chemistry. I have published more than 110 peer reviewed scientific papers, 20 invited reviews, 12 book chapters, and have given invited lectures in North America, Europe, and Japan.

I served lengthy terms as newsletter editor, first for the Canadian Association of Radiopharmaceutical Scientists (CARS) and later the UK Radiopharmacy Group, and a shorter term as News and Views editor for BNMS. I was chair of the Canadian Society of Nuclear Medicine and a member of the radiopharmacy committee of the European Association of Nuclear Medicine, the radioactive drugs committee of the British Pharmacopoeia, and the Administration of Radioactive Substances Advisory Committee. In the latter role I contributed to two reports on future provision of ^{99m}Tc. I represented the UK on a three person delegation to lobby the European Parliament during the drafting of the Clinical Trials Regulations.

My outside interests include music, theatre, and literature. In my retirement I intend to drink less coffee and more wine.

Development of Computers in Nuclear Medicine

18

E. David Williams

The story of computing in nuclear medicine is one of a role enabling continually improving performance and an interaction between technologies and applications, but sometimes with a pause for technical performance to catch up with user demand.

At the beginning of the medical use of radioactivity in clinical research and diagnosis, measurements of nuclear radiation, typically using a Geiger-Muller or a scintillation counter, enabled comparisons between the radioactivity of samples to be made. Subtraction of background was a simple arithmetical task, but calculation of ratios (for example to measure percentage uptake) required division, a more difficult task. It was made easy by use of an analogue computer system, the slide rule, which was a standard item of laboratory equipment until the early 1970s, when small portable electronic calculators replaced the mechanical and electromechanical calculators previously used for numerical calculation and made the slide rule redundant.

Before imaging became the dominant modality in the medical use of radioactivity, many research and clinical procedures had used radioactive tracers to study dynamic processes, typically the passage of a tracer substance through (for example) the kidneys. The countrate from a sodium iodide detector placed over a kidney would be used to drive the pen of a chart recorder to produce an activity-time curve then used to assess organ (e.g. renal) function. To separate the component due to uptake in the kidney from the decreasing contribution from activity in circulating blood, it was necessary to use a separate detector for the heart (blood pool) curve, and then subtract the blood data from the organ data by a process of deconvolution. This was a time-consuming task, while for other physiological investigations, there might be further physiological components to deal with and hence even more

E.D. Williams
Visiting Professor, Newcastle University (retired), Newcastle upon Tyne,
Tyne and Wear NE1 7RU, UK

© The Author(s) 2016
R. McCready et al. (eds.), *A History of Radionuclide Studies in the UK:
50th Anniversary of the British Nuclear Medicine Society*,
DOI 10.1007/978-3-319-28624-2_18

complexity. The task was, referred to as compartmental analysis of time-dependent data, and computers were applied to it in the 1960s. One type used was the analogue computer, which employed electronic components such as operational amplifiers and resistors, the connections between which could be altered with plug-in wiring, to model quantitatively the physiological compartments and produce an output signal which could be compared with the observed chart recording [1]. While this method was technically feasible, at the same time digital computers were becoming more generally available, and in the course of a few years they won this particular race and enabled also analysis of the uncertainties involved in fitting models to data [2]. Universities each generally had a mainframe computer which could be used if the data were presented in a suitable form. Initially, that could be an obstacle, with data having to be transferred to punched cards, but then in the late 1960s smaller, more accessible computers were installed in hospitals – the one I used at Hammersmith was installed to process pathology laboratory data, but fortunately was also available to other users. Like other installations at that time the computer was installed in a large air-conditioned room with several cabinets containing the central processor, magnetic tape drives, paper tape punch and reader, line printer and a teletype keyboard for controlling the computer. This computer had a central memory of 16 kB – about one million-fold less than that in a modern smart phone – giving some programming challenges for dealing with image data. By 1 970, interest had shifted from just analysis of organ uptake curves from separate small detectors to what was hoped would be more accurate results obtainable by acquisition and analysis of imaging data. My work at that time centred on use of a whole-body dual-detector rectilinear scanner equipped with a paper tape punch to record counts from each detector in every successive short time period. After getting the scan data into the computer, 'line printer' (paper) outputs were used in defining regions of interest and hence determine percentage organ uptake for research applications, including dosimetry for new radiotracers [3]. Meanwhile my colleague was using a specially built electronic system [4] for acquiring image data from the whole field of view of a gamma camera, in two-dimensional 64×64 frame mode, by conversion of the X, Y position data for each detected gamma ray using ADCs and two data buffers, acquiring into one while the other was read out onto magnetic tape which could then be taken to the London University computer centre This still left a fairly laborious process for defining regions of interest, but did enable analysis of dynamic studies simultaneously of multiple regions of interest, with tissue background activity correction.

The next step forward came from the advent of minicomputers in the 1970s, among which were for example the systems from Digital Equipment Corporation (DEC): the PDP-8 and later PDP 11. These were relatively small, and with magnetic disk drives and a colour monitor usually occupying just one or two 2 m tall equip-ment racks. They were dedicated systems for processing data acquired via ADCs from one gamma camera (and they cost about the same amount). The applications of these systems included measuring and correcting for gamma camera non-uniformity, renogram analysis, multiple ECG-gated cardiac bloodpool analysis (in which the patients ECG signal was used by the computer as a time marker enabling separate images for each phase of the cardiac cycle to be built up over several minutes) for measurement of left ventricular ejection fraction. In the early 1980s, gamma cameras capable of rotating the detector around the subject's body were developed and enabled single photon emission computed tomography [5], also using the dedicated computer. Initial applications included section imaging of the myocardium using thallium-201, bone and cerebral perfusion imaging, but adoption of section imaging generally grew quite slowly. At this time in the late 1970s/early 1980s positron emission (computed) tomography systems came into use initially for research, moving on into the 1990s to clinical diagnostic use, principally for staging cancer using F-18 FDG. As PET became more commonly used, technical advances using computer power followed similar paths to those for SPECT.

The computations for tomographic imaging initially required long processing times, but add-on parallel processing units could speed this up. Filtered back projection was the reconstruction technique used, as the potentially better iterative techniques would take too long. However in the 1990s ordered-subset expectation maximisation (OSEM) was developed and with the faster computers becoming available, that iterative reconstruction method has dominated in the 2000s [6]. So tomographic processing, by a more advanced technique, is now effectively instant, in comparison with the early lengthy procedures.

By about 1990 computing power was incorporated as an essential part of the standard gamma camera. Anger's resistor network design, at the heart of the gamma camera, was emulated digitally, using digital signal processors to collect and combine the photomultiplier tube outputs. Digital computing also quite dramatically improved the basic performance of the gamma camera through uniformity, linearity and energy corrections, while other corrections permitted the use of thinner detector crystals which improved spatial resolution. The console controlling data acquisition also typically provided a range of processing options. A separate additional computer system was however still popular as it gave some advantages, including continuity of use of processing software, in contrast to the built-in systems, when replacing the camera could mean changing how data were processed and presented. As computer power increased, a stand-alone computer could also acquire data from several cameras, using common systems for processing, archiving and output, providing images in standard formats.

Additional image data processing could attempt to correct for scatter radiation, collimator characteristics etc, and assess the performance of such techniques, as physical experimentation was increasingly replaced by computer simulations [7]. In clinical image processing applications, techniques were developed to define regions of interest automatically, and compare selected regions or whole images with standard image templates. However, while much work has been done on automated pattern recognition, these techniques are still usually seen as a support to a human reporter.

A clinical application of SPECT which has had a large impact is myocardial perfusion imaging, which brought closer involvement of cardiologists in nuclear medicine practice. The addition of ECG-gated SPECT brought a new, graphic dimension [8] which I think helped to sustain interest and helped to make SPECT a standard technique in most nuclear medicine services. In other clinical areas, cerebral perfusion and nigrostriatal SPECT extended clinical interest into the area of neuropsychiatry.

For clinical nuclear medicine, developments in the 2000s decade included the introduction of systems giving more integration of nuclear medicine in diagnostic imaging. One important area was the integration of tomographic image data (PET or SPECT) with structural imaging – initially CT and later also MRI, initially by computer techniques for co-registration of the images of structure and function, and later by integration of both functional and anatomical tomographic scanners: PET-CT, SPECT-CT and PET-MR. Another area of integration was PACS (picture archiving computer systems) which used common image data formats, or automated conversion between formats, and enabled digital images (now including all radiographic modalities, in addition to nuclear medicine) to be rapidly available across clinical data networks. Here there has been further integration, so the imaging specialist reporting on scans can now use a computer terminal and large display screens to review all relevant images, whatever the modality, and laboratory data, to dictate a report, using speech recognition software so that the text will be immediately available to clinicians.

References

1. Abrams ME, Crawley JCW, Green JR, Veall N. A comparative study of digital and analogue computer techniques for deconvolution procedures in clinical tracer studies. Phys Med Biol. 1969;14:225–32.
2. Glass HI, De Garreta AC. The quantitative limitations of exponential curve fitting. Phys Med Biol. 1971;16:119–30.
3. Williams ED, Merrick MV, Lavender JP. The distribution and dosimetry of In-lll bleomycin in man. Br J Radiol. 1975;48:275–8.
4. Vernon P, Glass HI. An off-line digital system for use with a gamma camera. Phys Med Biol. 1971;16:405–15.
5. Larsson SA. Gamma camera emission tomography. Development and properties of a multi-sectional emission computed tomography system. Acta Radiol Suppl. 1980;363:1–75.

6. Hutton BF. Recent advances in iterative reconstruction for clinical SPECT/PET and CT. Acta Oncol. 2011;50:851–8.
7. El Fakhri G, Buvat I, Benali H, Todd-Pokropek A, Di Paola R. Relative impact of scatter, collimator response, attenuation, and finite spatial resolution corrections in cardiac SPECT. J Nucl Med. 2000;41:1400–8.
8. Germano G, Kiat H, Kavanagh PB, Moriel M, Mazzanti M, Su HT, Van Train KF, Berman DS. Automatic quantification of ejection fraction from gated myocardial perfusion SPECT. J Nucl Med. 1995;36:2138–47.

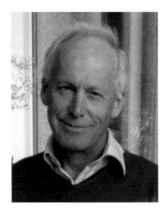

E. David Williams I decided on physics as my academic interest while at school. After graduation from Cambridge University in 1966, I started my career in Medical Physics in the radioisotope
section at Hammersmith Hospital headed by Harold Glass, learning about and contributing to
diagnostic and therapeutic services, and taking part in a variety of research projects. These involved
collaboration with haematologists, radiotherapists and radiologists. While there I was able to study
part-time at London University for an MSc and then completed a PhD on quantitative imaging –
analysis of scans to measure organ uptake of radioactivity. My wife and I decided in 1973 that
while our life in London had been interesting and enjoyable, we would like a change of scenery.
We drove from London to Calcutta, visiting interesting places en route, and then flew to New
Zealand. For 2 years I worked in the nuclear medicine department at Auckland Hospital during the
week, and enjoyed long sunny weekends. I returned to the UK to a university fellowship in neutron
activation analysis for body elemental composition medical research in Scotland. That group was
headed by Keith Boddy, who left a few years later to become head of the Regional Medical Physics
Department in Newcastle. His task was to expand clinical services across northern England. I took
the opportunity and challenge of setting up a new medical physics unit within RMPD and moved
to Sunderland in 1979. Initially providing a local nuclear medicine service, with one of the first
SPECT cameras in the UK, the unit grew beyond that to provide physiological measurement,
audiology, ultrasound and bone densitometry clinical services (and some clinical research), and
eventually moved into excellent new accommodation we designed at Sunderland Royal Hospital
in 2000. A sub-unit at South Shields opened in 1994 and another at Gateshead was added to my
unit a few years later. In 1992 I was appointed Regional Head of Nuclear Medicine Services,
responsible for leading and encouraging colleagues at all 13 hospital sites throughout the region of
north-east England and Cumbria towards providing high quality, up-to-date and efficient nuclear
medicine services. I think that together we made significant progress in that area. I enjoyed working with local medical, technical and scientific colleagues (including Sunderland University where
I was a visiting professor) and others across the UK and abroad through a variety of posts in professional bodies, including chair of publications at IPSM and Treasurer of BNMS. I also enjoyed
collaborating in research with colleagues from a wide range of specialties, in recent years involving imaging in dementia with John O'Brien at the Institute for Ageing and Health at Newcastle
University. I continued this work as visiting professor, using their PET-CT scanner for a project
that received funding just before my retirement from the NHS in 2009. The new 'leisure time'
enabled me to work on and complete the project over the next 5 years, and gave me more time for
my family and for the sporting activities I enjoy: ski-mountaineering, climbing and running.

E. David Williams

The Future Direction of Radiopharmaceutical Development

19

Philip J. Blower

The first use in humans of ^{24}Na-sodium chloride by Hamilton and Stone in 1936 [1] began a story in which ^{131}I-iodide became established for treating thyroid disease and radionuclide imaging became routine in hospitals. As important as the first commercial gamma camera (1968) [2] was the ^{99m}Tc generator, an elegantly simple device that solved the problem of world-wide distribution of a short half-life radionuclide, first used for medical purposes in 1961 [2]. A range of ^{99m}Tc-radiotracers quickly became available, including complexes of DTPA (renal function, lung ventilation), *meso*-DMSA (renal perfusion), bisphosphonates (bone), HIDA (liver) and various colloids (predating "nanotechnology" by decades) and macroaggregated albumin. They were easily synthesised in hospitals using simple kit vials, firmly establishing ^{99m}Tc as the staple medical radionuclide. They were largely serendipitous, arising from biological experiments using "off the shelf" chelating ligands selected without detailed knowledge of basic technetium chemistry [3], which was almost unstudied at that time. The simple preparation disguised extremely complex coordination chemistry. In most cases their structures remain unknown even now, and their approval in today's regulatory climate would have been most unlikely. Nevertheless they were extremely successful.

In the 1980s and 1990s, pioneered by leaders such as Davison and Deutsch, understanding of technetium chemistry grew [4] producing a new generation of tracers with a greater element of chemical design and with well-defined structures, but still with simple, kit-based labelling. The concept of technetium "cores" emerged – well-defined, stable complexes adapted to the coordination preferences of technetium, that could be functionalised for different purposes. Examples include the TcO^{3+} core (the basis of tracers such as MAG3 complex for renal function

P.J. Blower
Division of Imaging Sciences and Biomedical Engineering,
King's College London, St Thomas' Hospital, 4th Floor Lambeth Wing,
London SE1 7EH, UK

© The Author(s) 2016
R. McCready et al. (eds.), *A History of Radionuclide Studies in the UK:*
50th Anniversary of the British Nuclear Medicine Society,
DOI 10.1007/978-3-319-28624-2_19

imaging, "pentavalent" DMSA complex for medullary thyroid carcinoma and bone disease, HMPAO complex for cerebral perfusion imaging and cell labelling), $Tc(isonitrile)_6^+$ (sestamibi for myocardial perfusion imaging), TcO_2^+ (with tetraamine or diphosphine chelating ligands such as tetrofosmin), $Tc(CO)_3^+$ and $TcN(dithiocarbamate)_2$.

This set the stage for radiotracer design to shift towards targeting specific receptors and transporters, by incorporating ^{99m}Tc into peptides and proteins [3], and the term "molecular imaging" became both fashionable and relevant. It remained an important aspiration to synthesise ^{99m}Tc-radiopharmaceuticals via simple processes that are quick and use mild, aqueous conditions, avoiding the need for purification which adds undesirable complexity. However, ^{99m}Tc chemistry is complex, entailing both exchange of ligands and reduction of Tc(VII), and success has been limited. Radiolabelling procedures for biomolecules still involve multiple manipulations and poor specific activity. Hydrazinonicotinamide (hynic) and tricarbonyl ($Tc(CO)_3^+$) complexes come closest to achieving this, but both fall short and neither has led to commercial products. Due to a shift in commercial interests towards PET, very little effort has been devoted to this problem in the last decade and it remains a challenge to achieve "one-step" ^{99m}Tc biomolecule labelling.

Although emergence of positron emission tomography (PET) was roughly contemporaneous with that of the gamma camera, PET only became a routine clinical diagnostic tool in the 1990s, primarily driven by clinical use of the glucose analogue ^{18}F-fluorodeoxyglucose. The clinical adoption of PET demanded significant investment in infrastructure, requiring cyclotron installation within 2–4 h travelling distance of PET scanners. Availability of this costly new infrastructure spawned development of a much wider variety of PET tracers to enhance its versatility. Its better resolution and quantification made it increasingly attractive even for applications that do not require organic small molecules, creating roles for metallic positron-emitting radionuclides – ^{68}Ga, ^{89}Zr and copper isotopes $^{60/61/62/64}Cu$ – which, like ^{99m}Tc, are easier to use for proteins and peptides than ^{18}F and ^{11}C.

^{68}Ga (half-life 68 min) is rapidly emerging as "the new technetium" – a short half-life, generator-produced radiometal that is easily introduced into biomolecules. It produces a high positron yield and is readily chelated [5] with good kinetic stability. Despite growing clinical use, especially in Europe, the first commercial generator received marketing authorisation as recently as 2014. Although gallium chemistry is simpler than that of technetium (with only one relevant oxidation state (III)), the established chelating agents used to couple it to biomolecules require heating, low pH and purification steps, and have not been conducive to use in hospitals with limited radiochemistry facilities. A single-step, kit-based labelling procedure that works at room temperature, moderate pH and very low concentration would greatly increase its utility. Fortunately, considerable efforts have focused recently on developing new chelators to overcome these problems [5] and we will see their impact soon (Fig. 19.1).

Large biomolecules (e.g., monoclonal antibodies) with slow localisation and clearance require longer half-life tracers. The staple long half-life gamma-emitter has been ^{111}In, which can be attached to proteins using bifunctional chelators, usually DTPA and DOTA. A longer half-life "PET analogue" has inevitably emerged:

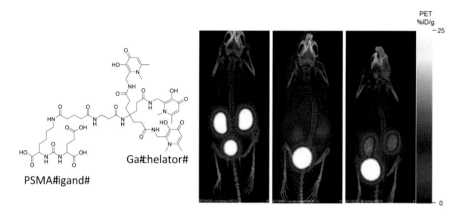

Fig. 19.1 PET-CT images of mouse bearing prostate-specific membrane antigen (*PSMA*) expressing prostate tumour (*left*), PSMA-expressing tumour (previously injected with a blocking dose of PSMA ligand) (*centre*), and PSMA-negative tumour (*right*), 1 h after injection of ^{68}Ga-labelled PSMA ligand conjugate of a tris(hydroxypyridinone) chelator (*left*) synthesised by a kit method at room temperature and pH 7 (Young J, Mullen GED, Blower PJ, 2015)

zirconium-89, and with desferrioxamine B as an effective bifunctional chelator for zirconium, [89]Zr PET has now been used to image the biodistribution and targeting of many antibodies ("immunoPET") in animal models and humans [6]. Longer-lived radionuclides can also usefully be incorporated into living cells to image their migration *in vivo*. Tracking leukocytes in this way using ^{111}In or ^{99m}Tc has been routine since the 1980s. A PET analogue would offer improvements in sensitivity, quantification and resolution suitable for new challenges in cell tracking emerging from the development of cell-based therapies and discoveries in cellular immunology. Indeed, the first [89]Zr cell labelling radiopharmaceuticals have been reported recently [7] (Fig. 19.2). Refinement in their chemistry, widespread preclinical and clinical application, and commercial availability may be anticipated in the coming years.

While ^{64}Cu has been widely studied in the last 20 years as a medium half-life positron emitter for biomolecule labeling, cell tracking and hypoxia imaging, it has begun to give way to alternatives. However its potential to study pathophysiological changes in copper trafficking (Fig. 19.3) in, for example, Wilson's disease, Menkes' disease, dementias (notably Alzheimer's), cancers and nutritional abnormalities [8] is now emerging. Similar possibilities are emerging to study other essential trace metals such as zinc (using [63]Zn) and manganese (using [52]Mn). This is a new field in which molecular imaging with radionuclides can make a major impact.

The combination of different imaging modalities that complement each other to overcome their individual limitations is a current trend. For example, while PET and SPECT have exquisite sensitivity (sub-picomolar concentrations in vivo) and provide truly "molecular" imaging, their resolution is poor. Magnetic resonance imaging (MRI), on the other hand, offers better anatomical resolution but large amounts of contrast agent are required, while optical imaging can be used at cell level [9] (unlike radionuclides and MRI) but is restricted in clinical use by poor tissue penetration. A new generation of scanners combining PET and MRI is now entering

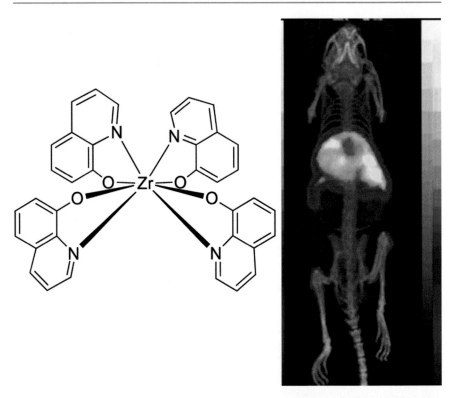

Fig. 19.2 Cell tracking with PET. PET-CT image of mouse 7 days after intravenous injection of 5T-33 myeloma cells labelled with [89]Zr tetrakis(oxinate), showing trafficking to liver, spleen and bone marrow (Ref. [7])

clinical use, driving new chemistry to produce combined modality contrast agents. For example, incorporating radionuclides into superparamagnetic iron oxide nanoparticles (SPION) allows combination of PET or SPECT with MRI. While particulate radiopharmaceuticals have been clinically used since the earliest days of nuclear medicine, the recent accumulation of capability in design, synthesis and characterisation of nanoparticles greatly enhances potential for multimodality imaging, albeit in specific niche areas such as imaging sentinel lymph nodes [10] (Fig. 19.4), reticuloendothelial system (liver, spleen, bone marrow), tumours (exploiting the enhanced permeability and retention effect), cell labelling and liposome-mediated drug and gene delivery.

In summary, the close cooperation of clinicians, physicists, engineers, biologists and chemists identifies capabilities, conceives challenges, discovers solutions and applies them in the clinic. Each discipline produces innovations that in turn drive innovations in the others. This is illustrated by the shift in the last decades from single photon radionuclide imaging towards PET, and in turn the

Fig. 19.3 PET-CT imaging of copper trafficking. Sagittal section (anterior at top of image) of mouse brain 30 min after injection of 64Cu-acetate, showing delivery to brain via choroid plexus. Left ventricle and fourth ventricle are indicated by *arrows* (Andreozzi, Bagunya-Torres, Blower, 2015)

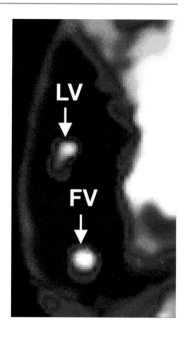

emerging shift from PET/CT towards PET/MRI and combination of these with optical imaging [9], which has led to new PET and combined modality radiopharmaceuticals. The next decade may see this recapitulated: the development of a new generation of gamma/SPECT scanners with resolution rivalling or exceeding that of PET will encourage renewed use and development of ^{99m}Tc tracers. The recently highlighted global fragility of ^{99m}Tc supply, far from foreshadowing the demise of ^{99m}Tc and SPECT, has stimulated renewed international effort to plan new reactors and cyclotron-based production, and develop new generator designs to cope with lower specific activity ^{99}Mo. This may soon stimulate a reversal in the recent decline of ^{99m}Tc chemistry research, producing innovations appropriate to the age of molecular imaging. New initiatives to develop a whole body PET scanner will stimulate increased use of short half-life radionuclides in combination (e.g., ^{82}Rb, ^{62}Cu, ^{13}N, ^{18}O) in a research setting, for metabolic characterisation of tissues in unprecedented detail by imaging multiple molecular targets in a single subject, again potentially in combination with MRI and MR spectroscopy. The arrival of cell-based therapies will bring improvements in use of radiopharmaceuticals for cell tracking, again using a multimodality approach. Conversely, the arrival of new, simple chemistry for ^{68}Ga may drive the installation of more PET scanners.

On a final optimistic note, there are hopeful signs that the adverse regulatory climate in the new millennium, which has held back the clinical and commercial translation of the wealth of new molecular imaging chemistry developed in the last 15 years, is at last becoming more amenable.

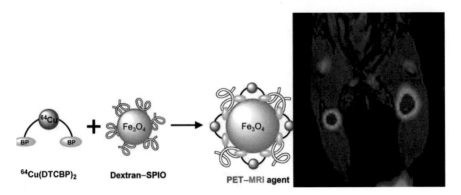

Fig. 19.4 Coronal PET-MRI image of mouse (*right*) after bilateral foot pad injection of ^{64}Cu-labelled iron oxide particles (*left*), showing transport to popliteal and iliac lymph nodes (Ref. [10])

References

1. Heilbron JL, Seidel RW. Lawrence and his laboratory: a history of the Lawrence Berkeley Laboratory. Berkeley: University of California Press; 1989.
2. Miale Jr A. Nuclear medicine: reflections in time. J Florida Med Assoc. 1995;82:749–50.
3. Blower PJ. A nuclear chocolate box: the periodic table of nuclear medicine. Dalton Trans. 2015;44:4819–44.
4. Dilworth JR, Parrott SJ. The biomedical chemistry of technetium and rhenium. Chem Soc Rev. 1998;27:43–55.
5. Price EW, Orvig C. Matching chelators to radiometals for radiopharmaceuticals. Chem Soc Rev. 2014;43:260–90.
6. Vugts DJ, Visser GWM, van Dongen G. Zr-89-PET radiochemistry in the development and application of therapeutic monoclonal antibodies and other biologicals. Curr Top Med Chem. 2013;13:446–57.
7. Charoenphun P, Meszaros LK, Chuamsaamarkkee K, Sharif-Paghaleh E, Ballinger JR, Ferris TJ, Went MJ, Mullen GED, Blower PJ. Zr-89 Oxinate(4) for long-term in vivo cell tracking by positron emission tomography. Eur J Nucl Med Mol Imaging. 2015;42:278–87.
8. Hueting R. Radiocopper for the imaging of copper metabolism. J Labelled Comp Radiopharm. 2014;57:231–8.

9. Fruhwirth GO, Diocou S, Blower PJ, Ng T, Mullen GED. A whole-body dual-modality radio-nuclide optical strategy for preclinical imaging of metastasis and heterogeneous treatment response in different microenvironments. J Nucl Med. 2014;55:686–94.
10. de Rosales RTM, Tavare R, Paul RL, Jauregui-Osoro M, Protti A, Glaria A, Varma G, Szanda I, Blower PJ. Synthesis of Cu-64(II)-Bis(dithiocarbamatebisphosphonate) and its conjugation with superparamagnetic iron oxide nanoparticles: in vivo evaluation as dual-modality PET-MRI agent. Angew Chem Int Ed. 2011;50:5509–13.

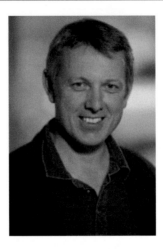

Philip J. Blower Since 2006 Phil Blower has been at King's College London as Chair in Imaging Chemistry in the Division of Imaging Sciences and Biomedical Engineering. As Head of the Imaging Chemistry and Biology Dept., he has built a large interdisciplinary research group with wide interests covering radiopharmaceutical chemistry and biology for PET, SPECT and radionuclide therapy, including a continuing focus on copper radionuclides (especially in hypoxia imaging) as well as technetium, rhenium, gallium, fluorine and more recently gallium and zirconium. He is PI or co-PI on current grants worth about £25 m, including a Cancer Research UK/EPSRC Cancer Imaging Centre, a Wellcome/EPSRC Medical Engineering Centre, and an EPSRC Doctoral Training Centre in Medical Imaging. He has published more than 150 peer-reviewed papers and supervised more than 28 successful PhD students. He has served on various peer review panels for international grant awarding bodies and journals and as Editor in Chief of Nuclear Medicine Communications. His path to this point followed a BA in Natural Sciences (Cambridge) and DPhil in Chemistry (Sussex), and postdoctoral experience in inorganic chemistry at Indiana University and Oxford University. His first academic post was a joint appointment at Kent and Canterbury Hospital (Radiopharmacy) and the University of Kent (Biosciences), where he combined the two roles to develop a number of new radiopharmaceuticals for imaging and therapy, including the earliest clinical evaluation of Re-186 and Re-188 targeted therapeutic radiopharmaceuticals and pioneering use of copper radionuclides for PET in Europe.

A Personal Reflection

20

Tom Nunan

> *Why on earth are you doing that – the specialty will be dead in*
> *a few years, now that we have CAT scanning.*

This is what I heard in the late 1970s when I studied for the MSc in Nuclear Medicine. At that time there was only planar imaging and most of the imaging work was brain, liver and bone scanning largely for metastases and lung scans for pulmonary emboli. (For the purposes of this paper I will not cover thyroid work which has really not changed that much.) The bone scans were taken on a rectilinear scanner which technically had a better resolution than the gamma camera, but was slow and produced images that did not look anatomical so were not liked by clinicians. This is the same problem that ultrasound had, especially in the early days, when the clinicians could not understand the images (assuming they were available).

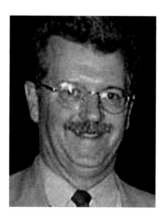

T. Nunan
Nuclear medicine, St Thomas' Hospital,
First floor, Lambeth Wing, Westminster Bridge Road, London SE1 7EH, UK

© The Author(s) 2016
R. McCready et al. (eds.), *A History of Radionuclide Studies in the UK:*
50th Anniversary of the British Nuclear Medicine Society,
DOI 10.1007/978-3-319-28624-2_20

CT brain scanning had been around since 1971. I did what were then called House Physician and Surgeon jobs at the West Middlesex Hospital in West London and I remember well the CT scanner (the first in the world) at the nearby Atkinson Morley Hospital. Quickly everyone realised the potential in diagnosis for brain diseases (not too surprising when one considers that it replaced such invasive procedures as air encephalography) and within a few years the role of CT brain scanning was established. I later looked at the early history of Xrays for an exhibition at Guy's and was struck by the similarity between the rapid rate of adoption of Xrays (Roentgenograms in those days but changed in the First World War to Xrays and Roentgengraphy changed to Radiology). But I digress.

CT brain scanning eventually replaced radionuclide blood-brain barrier scanning. In those days the resolution of everything was too poor for imaging techniques to be used for dementia. There was also the growing development of ultrasound which was to replace liver scanning, again used mainly for detecting metastases. So up went the cry that Nuclear Medicine had no future. Well, along came thallium cardiac imaging. I remember in around 1985 comparing workloads over the decade and the number of studies performed had increased, despite losing all the liver and brain scans, largely as a result of the cardiac work. In addition as an indicator of what was to come, the complexity of studies was increasing. With this came a small but useful technological advance, what were called 'large' field of view cameras. Now routine, but what it meant is it was now possible to image the whole of the chest and get in the shoulders in one image. This resulted in images which referring clinicians found easier to interpret – those of you who are still following my gist will see a trend here. Those of you who are not – well never mind!

Then along came whole body CT. (The first scanner was made by EMI and was thus called an Emiscan, then when other manufacturers entered the fray they were called CAT scans and at later date this was shortened to CT – why? I don't know). Whole body CT imaging developed in the late 80's and St Thomas' had, I believe, the second whole body EMI scanner. Again people worried that Nuclear Medicine had no future. In contrast to the CT brain scanner the use of whole body CT took some time to establish itself. I think this is because it was slow and the images were degraded by movement artefacts. Of course the first demonstration of Computerised Tomography by Oldendorf in 1961 was using isotopes and it was not developed further because the rest of technology for imaging was not ready. (Another digression, if we were to go back to 1890 and asked what do we want to develop, a functional imaging methodology for the body or 'shadow' images, which would we choose? It was only the ease with which Xray apparatus could be made and the lack of such technology that resulted in Roentgenography taking on the leading role in imaging).

Then along came SPECT. (I always wondered why do we have SPECT but not TCT or PECT?) SPECT was a bit a a game changer in cardiac studies since one now had the heart imaged in a way the cardiologists could understand and the result was a huge expansion in our cardiac workload to the point that full list cardiac studies were being performed 3–4 days per week, as opposed to one small list every 2 weeks. SPECT cardiac studies took off despite there being little evidence that they had better accuracy than planar images, because of the improvement in image perception. Again to digress, I remember clearly in the late 80s, we were asked to do a thallium scan on a lady. This was a very unusual occurrence indeed. Over the years equality arrived and possibly overshot since when I retired it was my impression that female cardiac requests outnumbered male.

One of the factors that helped to develop cardiac scanning was the discovery that with conventional imaging protocols, myocardium that did not take up Thallium could be shown to be viable post revascularisation rather than as conventional wisdom had it, infarcted. Indeed I remember cardiac surgeons saying as much but a paper in the NEJM showed these anecdotes to be correct. The above statement might sound counterintuitive but the threat this raised resulted in two things happening. The first was to relook at the thallium protocol. It was then realised that the one day protocol with a stress image first and a redistribution image several hours later was a compromise between convenience, dose and accuracy. The correct way to do the study was to have a proper rest image. This leads to the second point which was that thallium for a 2 day injection protocol had a rather high radiation dose. Thus the manufacturers developed ^{99m}Tc tracers to do the job. This had an added advantage since modern cameras are made with ^{99m}Tc in mind and are more suited to ^{99m}Tc than Tl^{201}. To yet another digression, it is always useful to look at things from the basics, often there are compromises made which will always result in sacrificing something. I am reminded of the endless papers on the measurement of GFR where there was (and maybe still is) compromise in the number of samples taken versus the convenience to the patient.

Things got quiet then in terms of development, MRI was coming on the scene, CTPA was supposed to replace lung scanning. Yet again the cry went up – 'Nuclear Medicine has no future'. Perhaps it is this threat that gets people looking hard at what they do and coming up with advances.

But to counter MRI we had PET scanning then PET/CT. The real development that allowed these to happen was the development of computer power. Many of those of us who are 'more senior' will remember stories of studies being performed, the data loaded into the computer and then everyone went home for the night and if they were lucky it would be ready to look at in the morning. I also remember the South-East region getting some gamma cameras which could either acquire an image or process it, not both at the same time. Think how it is now – even the most complex PET/CT study is ready before the patient leaves the room.

I think we are eventually arriving at a point where the advantages of functional imaging are becoming main stream, all as a result of hybrid images and the excellent image quality that they provide. Our referring clinicians can easily interpret the images to see and more to the point, understand what we are talking about in the report. (Beware of my predictions, I once was asked by GE what I thought of double headed cameras and said I thought they were too expensive for people to buy. But as was once said "All technology is too expensive." When I looked on Google to see who said this, I could not find it, but I note that UEFA President Platini is saying it in relation to goal line cameras, so it is bound to come).

So over my career, Nuclear Medicine changed out of all recognition. Few of the types of study that I started with are routine now, they have either been replaced by other imaging modalities (liver scans), been significantly modified (SPECT bone and lung scans) or are completely new (sentinel node and PET/CT). Thus although people may say again 'don't consider Nuclear Medicine as a career because it will not last' – they are and have been wrong!

Printed in the United States
By Bookmasters